# 104 Ways to Starve Your Anger and Feed Your Soul

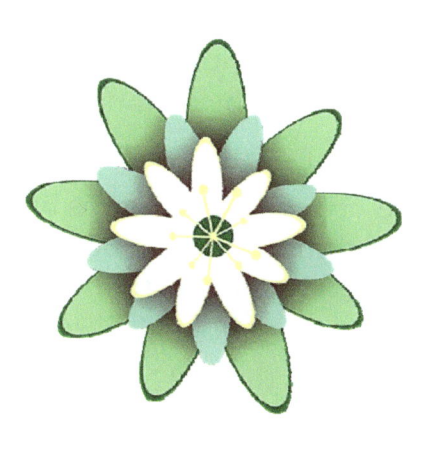

Robyn Wheeler

# 104 Ways to Starve Your Anger and Feed Your Soul

Robyn Wheeler

**DISCLAIMER:**

Before considering any technique described herein as a form of physical, mental or emotional treatment, the author recommends that you seek the advice of a qualified physician or professional therapist.

Published by
Born Mad, LLC
Post Office Box 1783
Mabank, Texas 75147-1783
www.bornmad.org

Content Editing by Pearl Cantrell
Copyediting by Lynette Smith
Cover Design by Victoria Vinton

Copyright © 2013 Robyn Wheeler

All rights reserved. No part of this book may be reproduced or transmitted in any form or by any means without written permission from the publisher.

ISBN (Paperback): 978-0-615-69450-4
Library of Congress Control Number: 2012921054

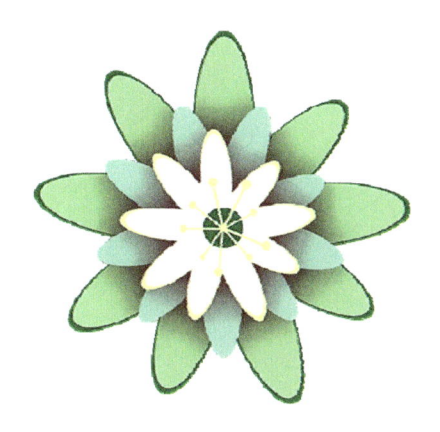

Dedicated to those who struggle with anger,
the underlying emotions that cause it
and the hopelessness anger can create.
May you find love, peace
and happiness.

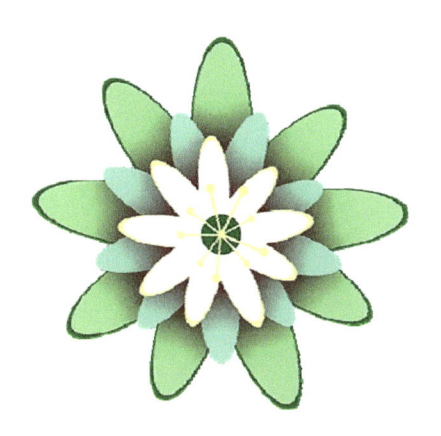

For every minute you are angry, you lose
60 seconds of happiness.

*–Author Unknown*

# Contents

Foreword .................................................................ix

Acknowledgments ...............................................xi

Introduction ..................................................... xiii

104 Ways to Starve Your Anger
    and Feed Your Soul........................................1

Prayers .............................................................107

Related Resources.............................................111

About the Author .............................................113

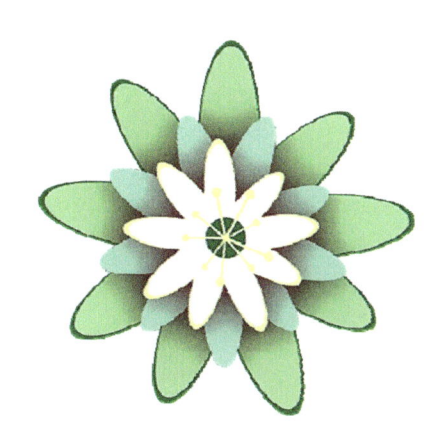

# Foreword

I once saw a billboard which read "The person who angers you, controls you." Unless you are a robot, with no internal emotional circuits, the content within this book will greatly affect your heart.

Although short in words but long in meaning, the message from each page is inspiring and encouraging. I highly credit my friend, Robyn Wheeler, for her producing in written form, messages of hope and healing to hearts that have been damaged by anger. It is awesome to see the spark of Robyn's spirit shine in moments of darkness.

To Robyn and her husband, Ron, I thank them both for their inspiration.

**Father Dan Daugherty**
Pastor and Friend
St. Jude Catholic Church
Gun Barrel City, Texas

# Acknowledgments

Thank you to my husband, Ron, for your constant support, encouragement and love.

To my friend and editor, Pearl Cantrell of *The Monitor of Cedar Creek Lake*, thank you for your patience, time and excellence in editing.

To my friend and copyeditor, Lynette Smith of All My Best, thank you for being a part of my growth. Your astute advice is greatly appreciated.

To Victoria Vinton of Coyote Press, thank you for your beautiful cover design and advice on how to make this project come together.

To Father Dan Daugherty, thank you for accepting us into your world and giving of your kindness and thoughtfulness.

To Carol Saucedo, thank you for your friendship and review of this work.

To all my family members, I love you and wish you an eternity of peace and happiness.

To my readers, thank you for your support. I wish you an anger-free, peaceful life.

To God, without whom none of this would have been possible, my life is better, happier and healthier with You guiding the way.

# Introduction

One cannot look outside oneself to overcome anger. The only way to live an anger-free life is by changing what is in the inside.

Most people blame others or unfortunate events for their anger. The truth is you are the only one responsible for your anger. No one makes you mad. You allow yourself to get mad and then act on those emotions.

*104 Ways to Starve Your Anger and Feed Your Soul* brings awareness to the emotions beneath the anger such as fear, shame, embarrassment, guilt, and insecurities, and shows you various techniques to rid yourself of these thoughts.

Anger is a hindrance to a happy, fulfilling and peaceful life. When you change your thoughts and perception of everything around you, anger will no longer control your life.

**Robyn Wheeler**

# 104 Ways to Starve Your Anger and Feed Your Soul

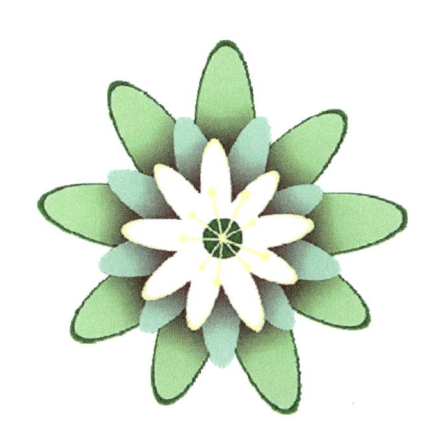

# 1

Take time to relax every day, even if only for a few minutes. Breathe deeply and slowly, allowing calm to take over. Calmness will override angry feelings.

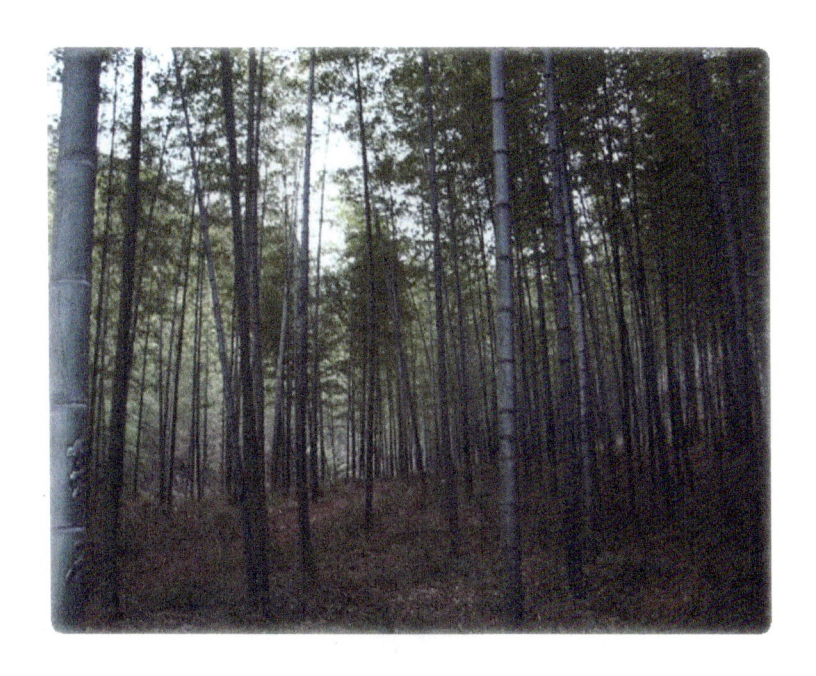

# 2

Happiness is not an inanimate object that can be purchased from a store. Happiness is located within you. Only you have the power to make yourself happy. Happiness is a state, not a destination.

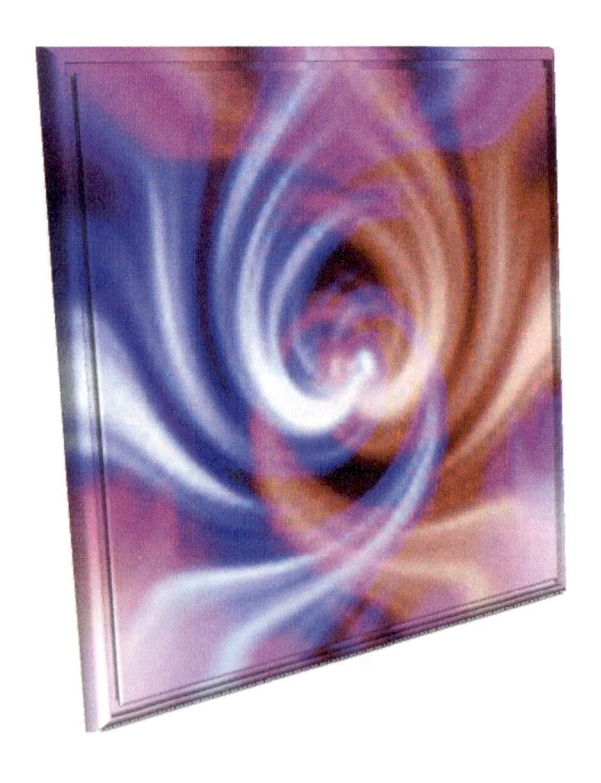

# 3

Know that whatever problem you have will not last forever. The solution will appear at the right time, in the right order and in a way that is just right for you. When faced with a problem, don't get mad; instead, ask questions, find out all you need to know about the situation and then look for a solution before making a decision.

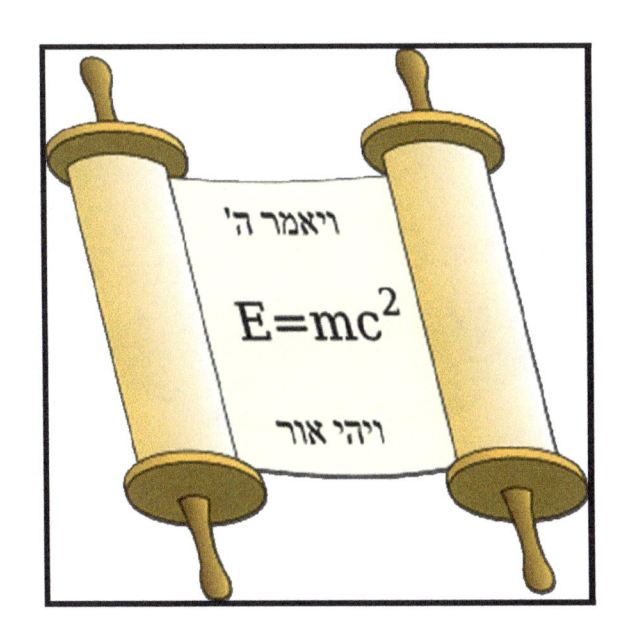

# 4

Find delight in the little things such as a young baby learning to walk, the smell of a beautiful flower or soaking in a warm tub. Remind yourself daily to enjoy the small things, for they are the big things in life.

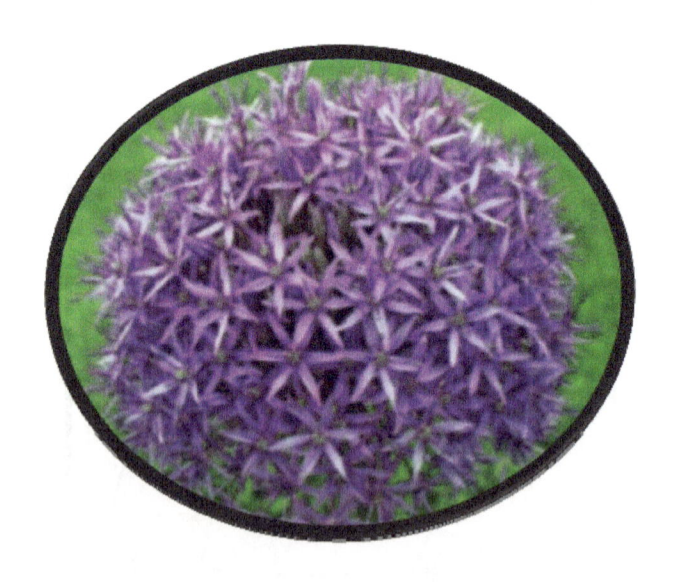

# 5

Say daily affirmations to defuse the stress and anxiety in your life. Having confidence in yourself will lessen angry feelings.

> Whether you think you can,
> Or you think you can't,
> You're right.
>
> -Henry Ford

# 6

Try to love everyone, no matter what they do that you may dislike. If you love at all times, you will find happiness within yourself. Dislike the deed, not the one who acted out the deed.

## LOVE

Is patient and kind

Does not envy or boast

Is not proud, rude or self-seeking

Is not easily angered

Keeps no record of wrongs

Does not delight in evil

Rejoices with the truth

Always protects, trusts, hopes

Always perseveres

And never fails.

*I Corinthians 13:4-7, 13*

# 7

Avoid striving for perfection. Love yourself and others despite imperfections. Attempting to be perfect is self-defeating and creates a no-win situation. A no-win situation is a breeding ground for anger.

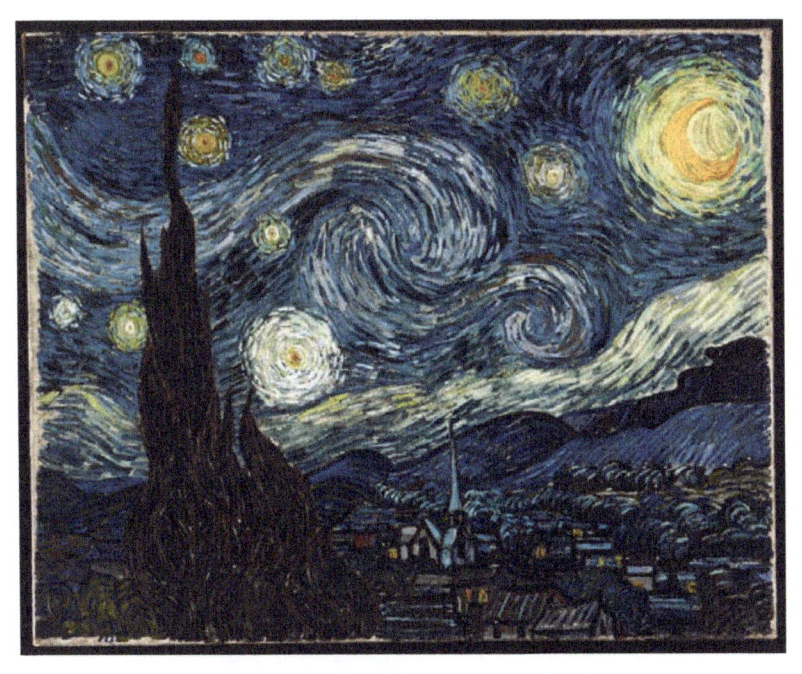

Starry Night, *Vincent Van Gogh*
*Dutch Post-Impressionist Painter*
*1853–1890*

# 8

Accept what is. There will be many things throughout your life that you cannot change. Accept the good with the bad. Getting angry over things you cannot change is futile.

> **If you don't like something, change it.
> If you can't change it, change the way you think about it.**

# 9

Incorporate change in your life. If you are stagnant, you'll go nowhere. If you change, you'll move ahead. Believe in change for a happier, more fulfilling life.

> Change is the essence of life; be willing to surrender who you are for what you could become.
>
> -Author unknown

# 10

Fear creates anger. Force yourself to make decisions based on facts, not irrational fears. Even scary things are good in their own unique way.

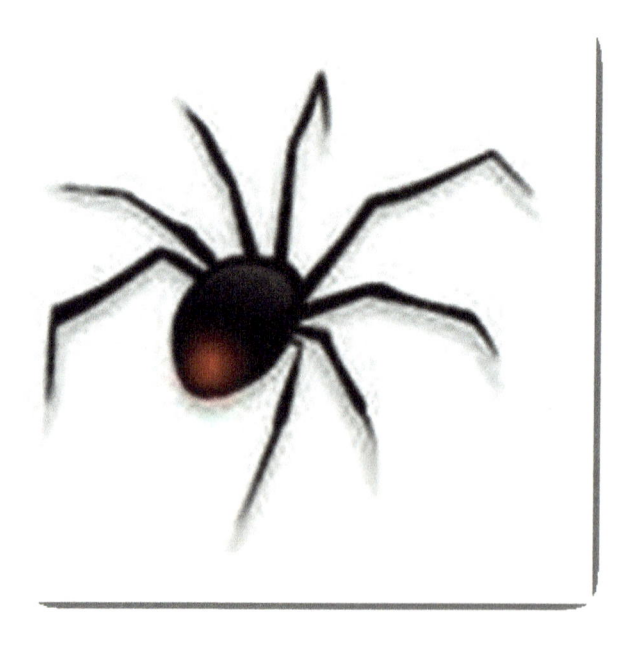

# 11

Learn to fail. Love your failures as mistakes and imperfections. This will allow you to grow and become a better person. The most successful people in history all learned to fail.

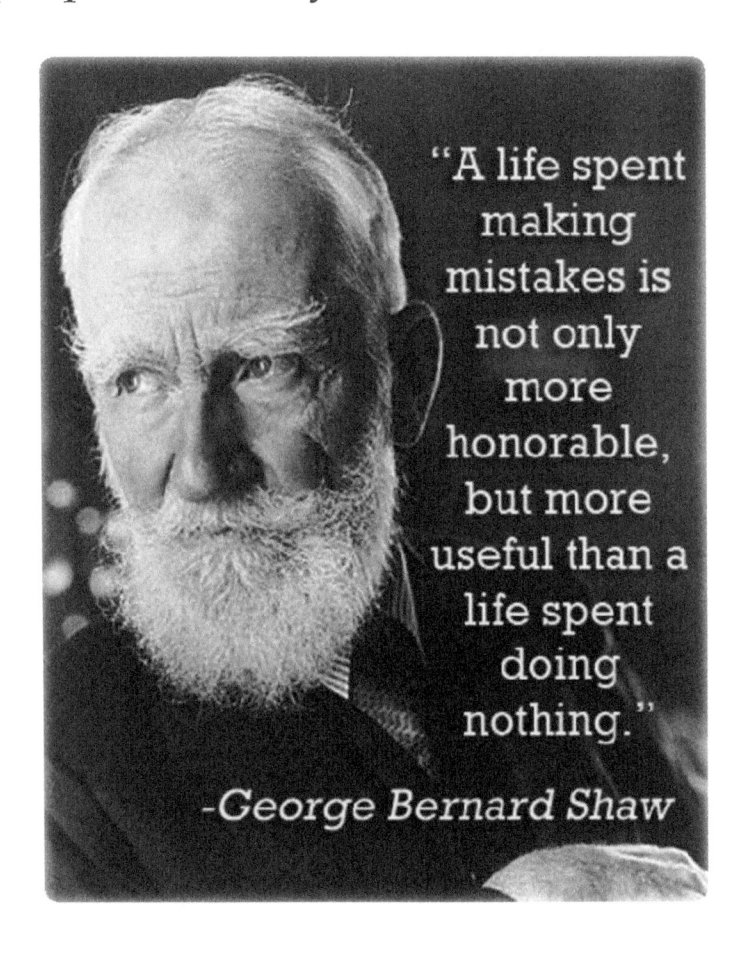

"A life spent making mistakes is not only more honorable, but more useful than a life spent doing nothing."

-George Bernard Shaw

# 12

Being angry takes more energy than being happy. Put your energy towards peace and happiness. It will be less exhausting.

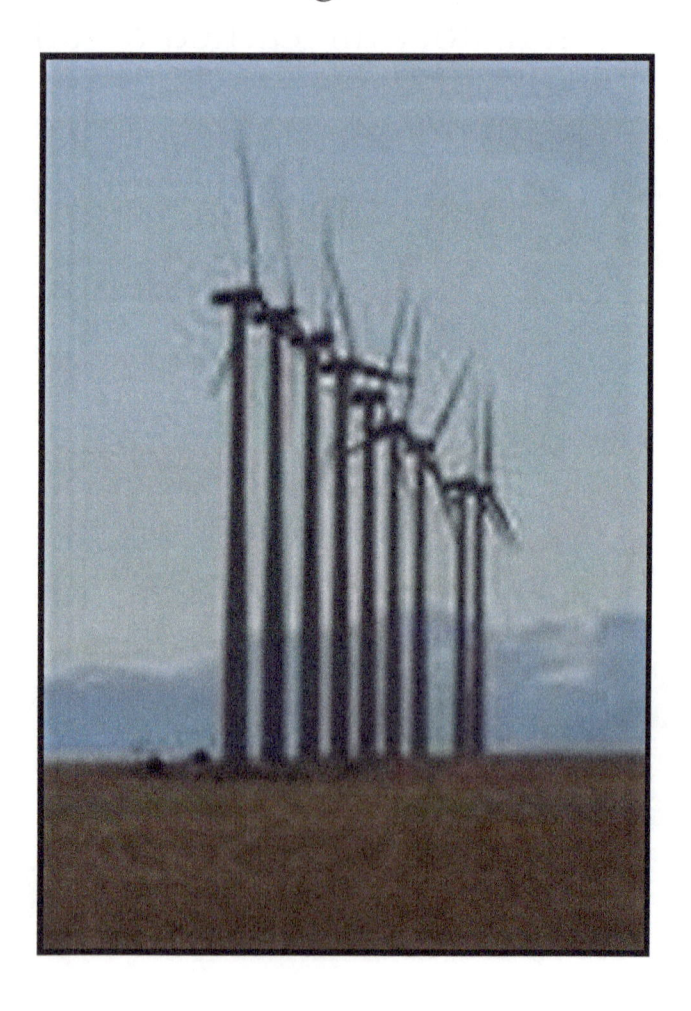

# 13

Know that you are not in control. A Higher Power is in control. Being mad because of circumstances is equal to being mad at your Creator.

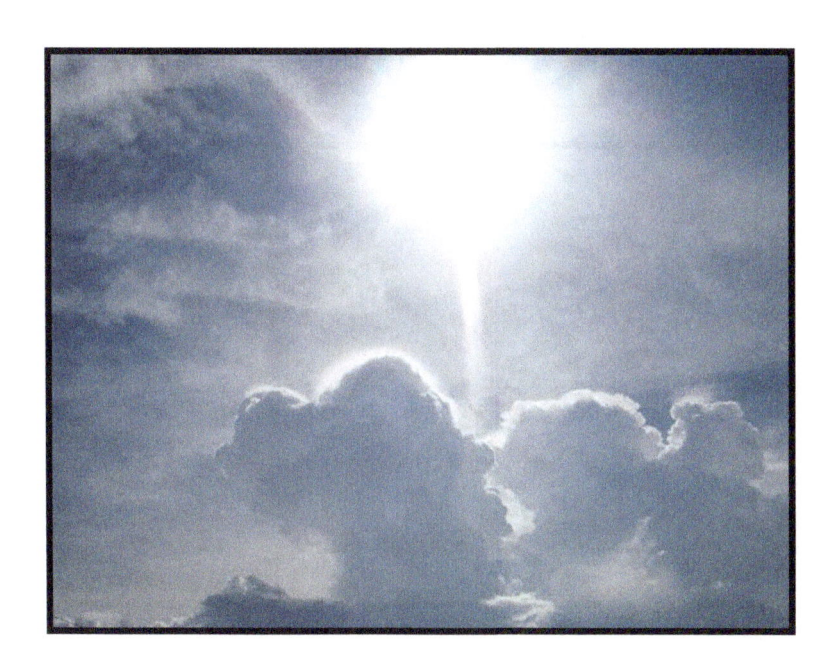

# 14

Rigidity causes anger. Flexibility creates happiness. When you insist all things must go your way, you set yourself up for anger. Learn mental flexibility.

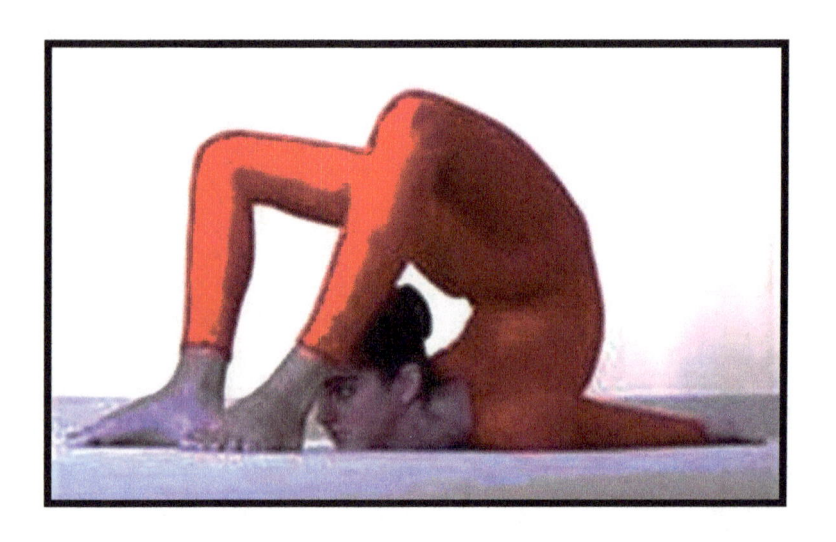

# 15

Know that there is always something good on the other side of something bad. There is a silver lining behind the dark cloud.

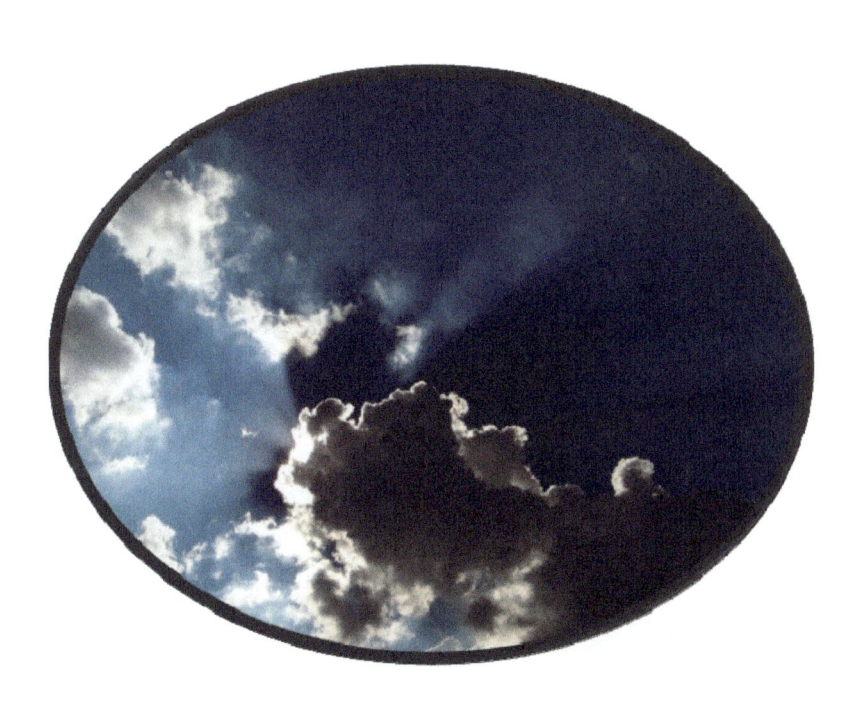

# 16

Avoiding mental and physical pain is not possible. Know that pain is a fact of life. What matters is how you deal with it and what you learn from it.

> Learning is a gift.
>
> Even when pain is your teacher.

# 17

Practice random acts of kindness toward a stranger every day. Helping others will create happiness within you, thus ending your anger.

> DON'T WAIT FOR PEOPLE TO BE KIND, SHOW THEM HOW.
> -AUTHOR UNKNOWN

# 18

Anger pulls you away from Spirit. Forgiveness pushes you toward Spirit. Find the gentle Spirit within you.

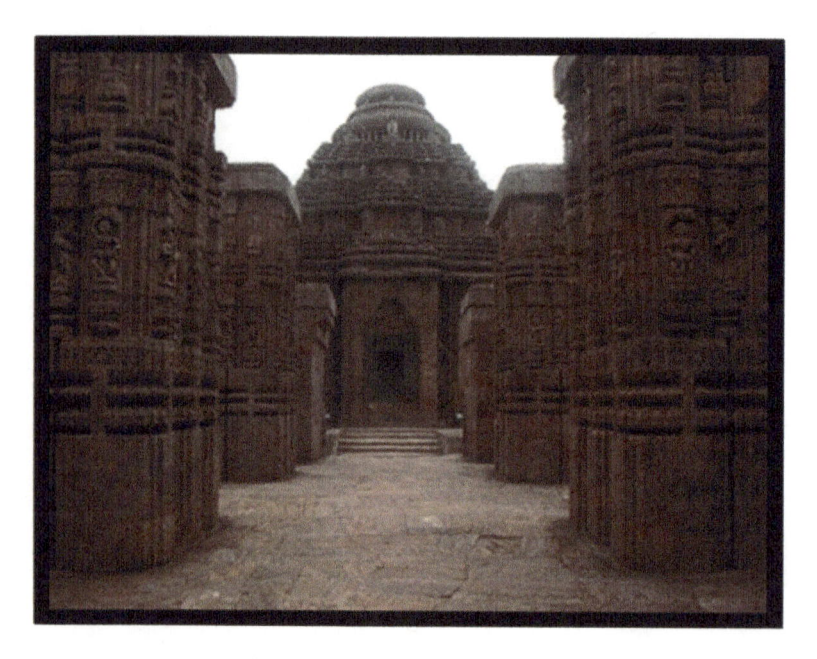

*Konark Sun Temple, Orissa, India*

# 19

Avoid exaggerating your current situation. No one enjoys being around a drama queen, and you'll only make yourself believe your situation is worse than it really is. Avoid making a mountain out of a molehill.

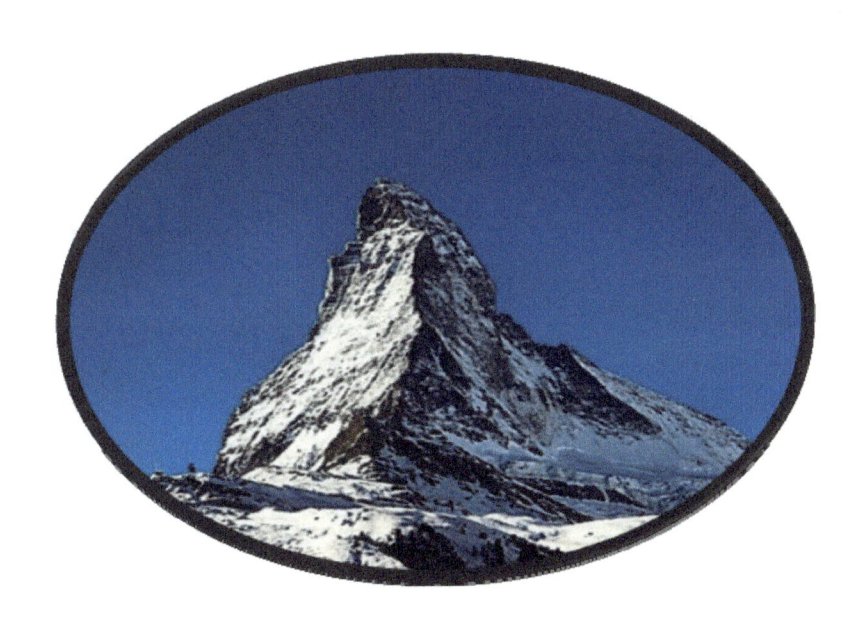

# 20

If you make a decision when you are angry, you will most likely make the wrong choice. Remember, you cannot take back what you say or do.

> **I am who I am today because of the choices I made yesterday.**
> *- Eleanor Roosevelt*

# 21

Peace is never controlling. Anger will keep you in shackles forever. Don't allow anger to run your life.

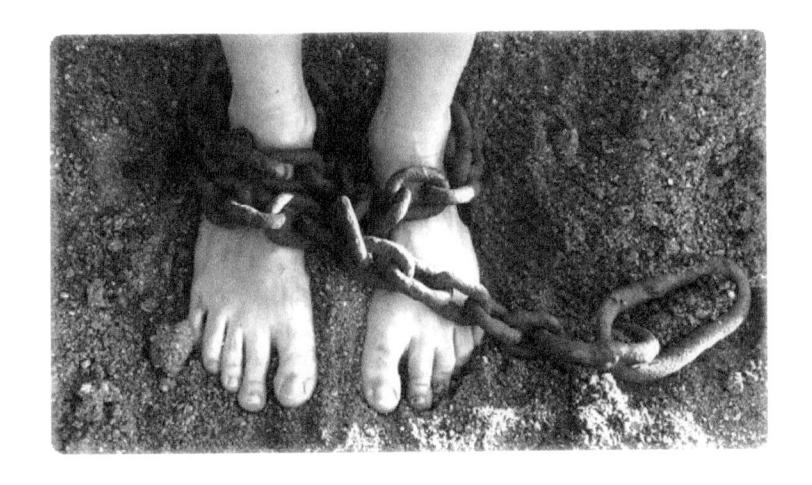

# 22

The key to happiness lies within your reaction to events, not the events themselves. You can decide how to feel.

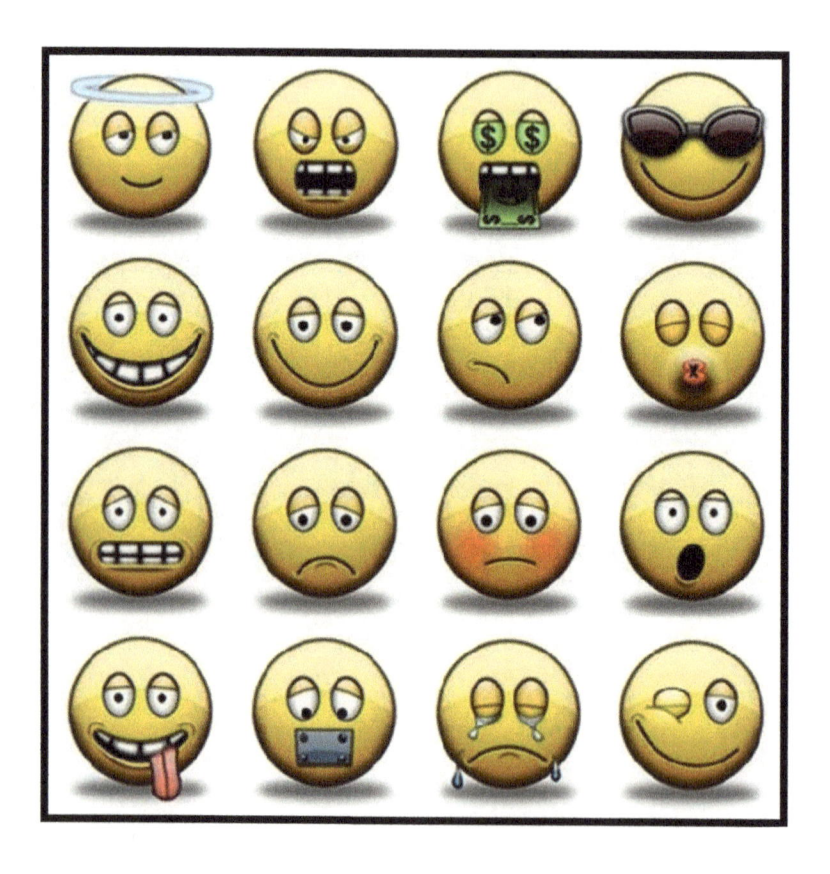

## 23

Sulking or walking around in silence will not improve a situation; it will only make it worse. Don't go from bad to worse. Go from bad to better.

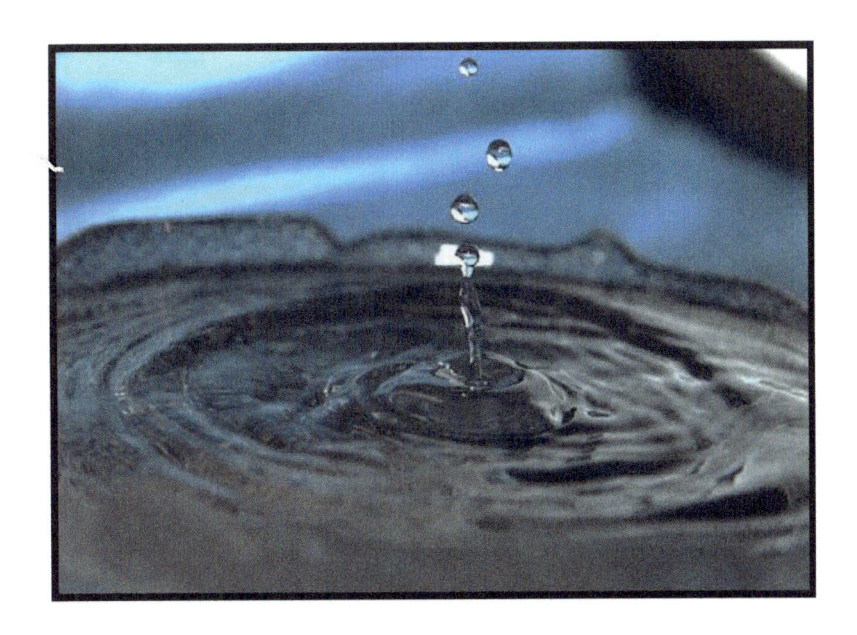

# 24

Forgive everyone for everything. Resentment creates unhappiness within your soul and spirit. You cannot live anger free if you are unwilling to forgive yourself as well as others.

*Hanging onto resentment is letting someone you despise live rent-free in your head.*

–Ann Landers, American Advice Columnist, 1918–2002

# 25

Eliminate the word "should" from your vocabulary. No one can do something differently after it's already been done. Saying someone "should" do something is futile. Believing something "should" be different creates anger and resentment.

> **INSANITY IS DOING THE SAME THING OVER AND OVER, EXPECTING DIFFERENT RESULTS.**
>
> **- ALBERT EINSTEIN**

# 26

Your ego contributes to your madness. Avoid allowing vanity, pride and self-absorption to dictate your actions.

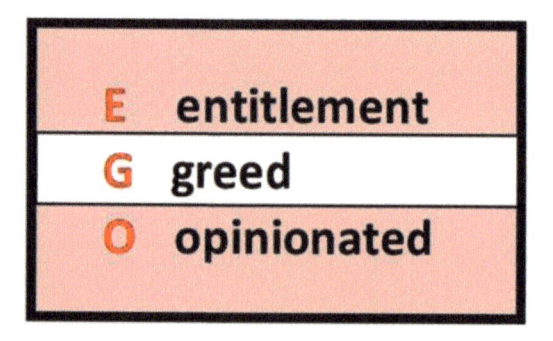

| E | entitlement |
|---|---|
| G | greed |
| O | opinionated |

> The best lesson of life is to listen and learn from everyone, because *nobody knows everything* and everybody knows something.

# 27

Be willing to do anything to get rid of your anger. What can it hurt to try something new?

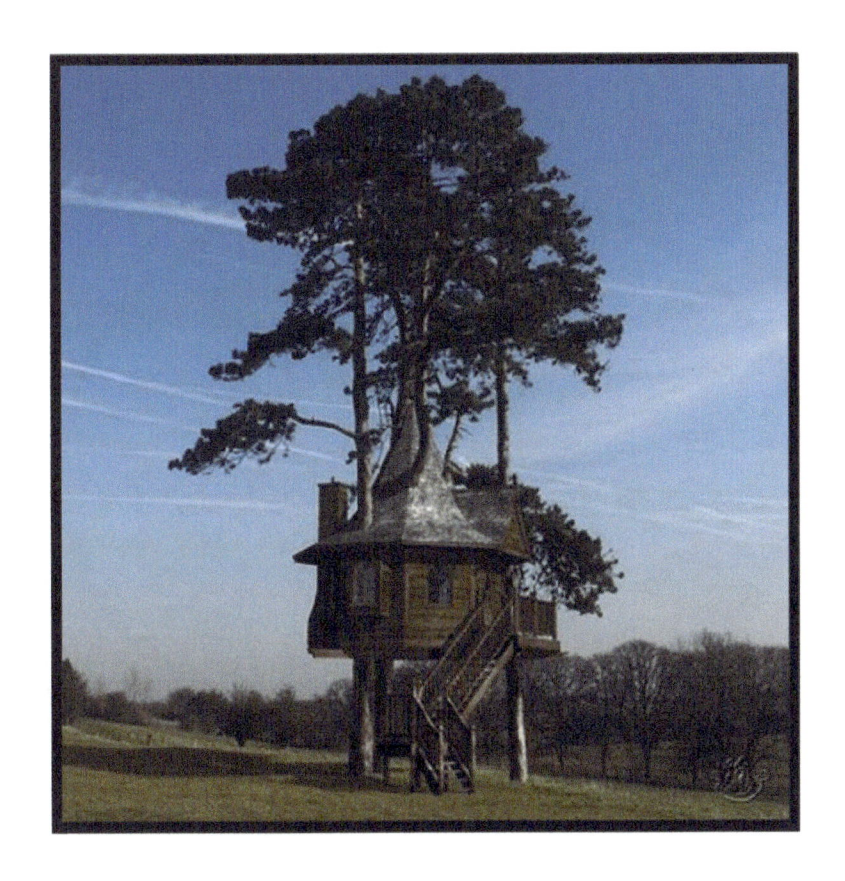

# 28

Anger can be addictive, just like drugs, alcohol or food. To break the anger cycle, heal anger by treating it like an addiction.

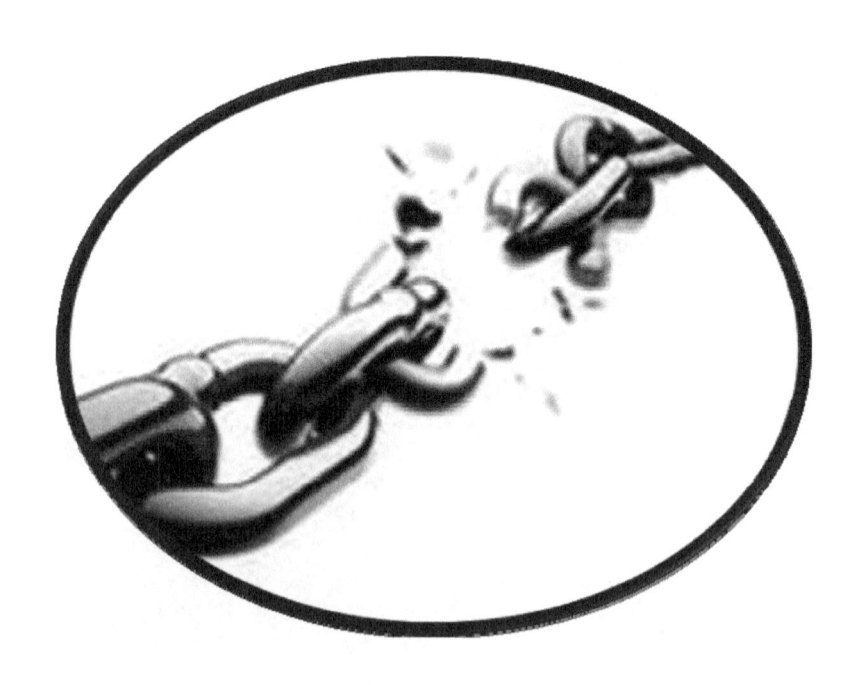

## 29

Being closed-minded creates anger. Avoid judging others to prevent madness. Remember, things aren't always as they seem.

> **Judging others does not define who they are.**
>
> *It defines who you are.*

# 30

Handle the moment the best you know how. Enjoy today, as tomorrow is still a day away. Each sunrise provides an opportunity to do things differently.

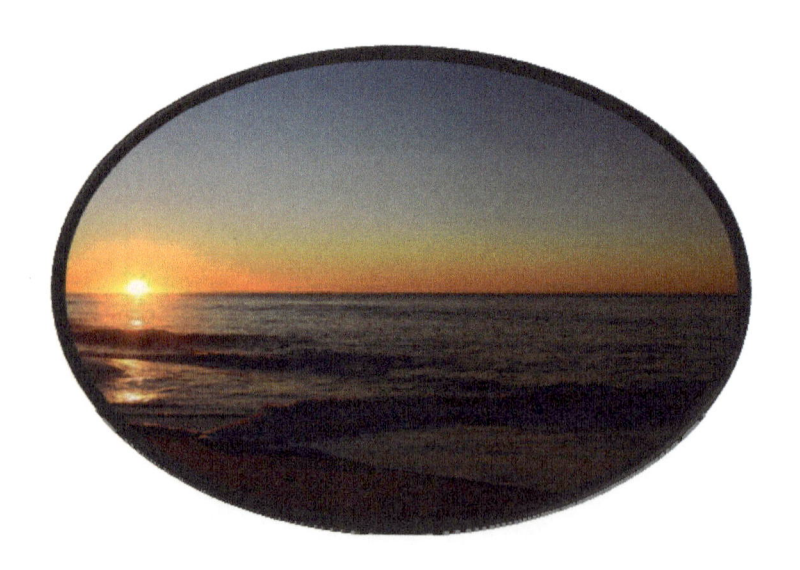

# 31

Avoid name calling, berating others and creating chaos. These things will not bring peace or happiness. When you call others names, you make yourself look bad. Say kind words, even about others you may not particularly like.

> If you cannot say anything nice, don't say anything at all.

# 32

If it seems you are mad at most everyone, you are really mad at yourself. Take what you are complaining about and figure out how it fits into your actions, thoughts and feelings. Then take steps to repair the damage.

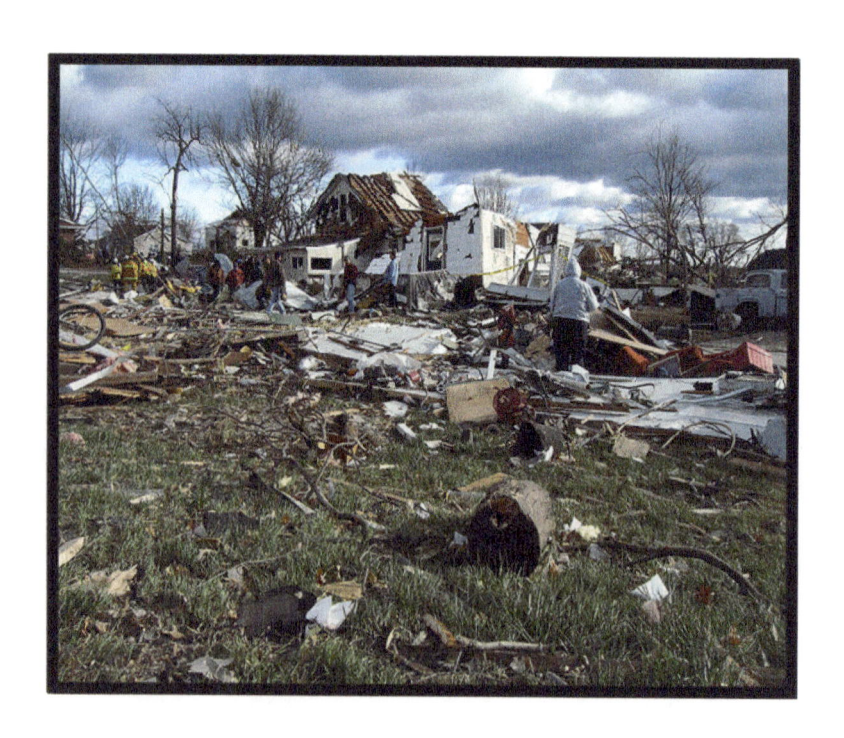

## 33

Remember, it's all small stuff. And there is never a good reason to be mad over the small stuff. Every day of life is like a grain of sand. Eventually, you will end up creating a beautiful beach.

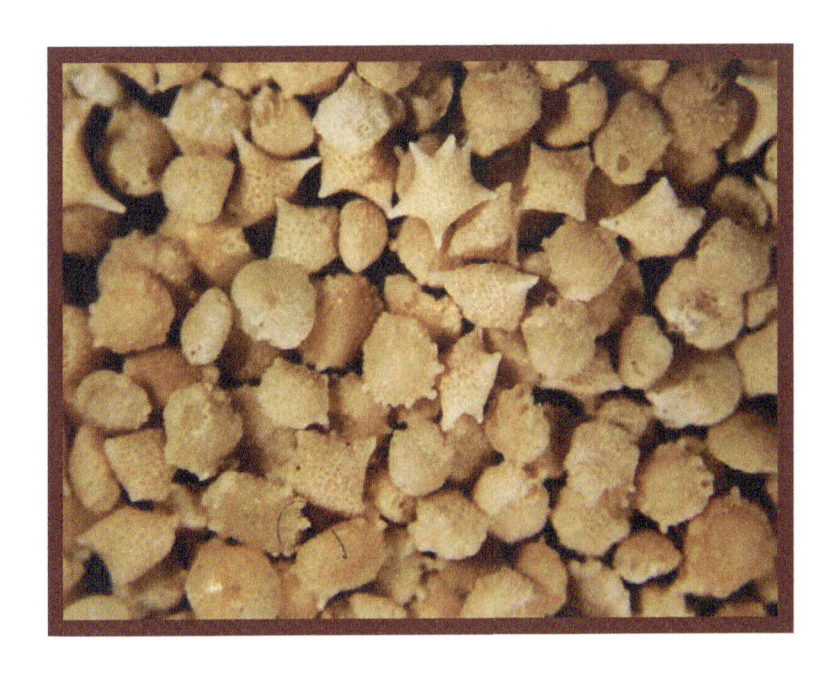

# 34

Anger is like fire. If you don't put it out quickly, its damage will spread quicker and further out. Don't char the good things in life.

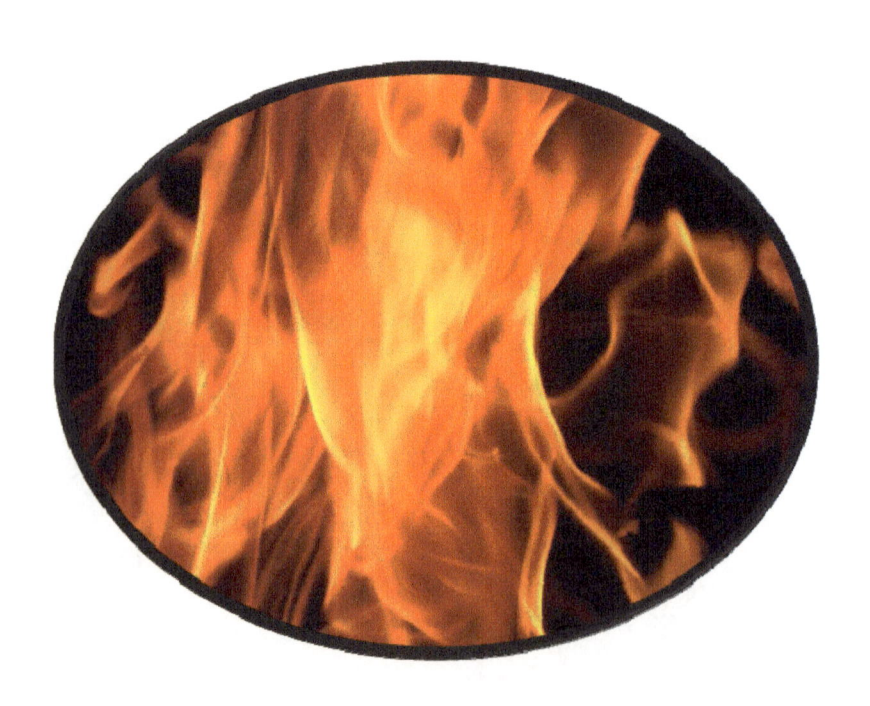

# 35

Anger is pointless. Remind yourself on a daily basis to create something good and amazing that will make a difference in someone else's life.

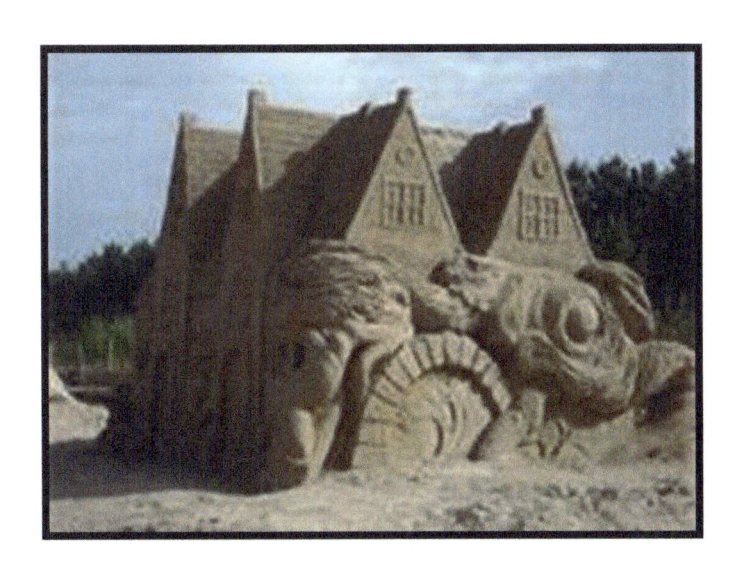

# 36

Give someone a compliment every day – it will make both of you feel better.

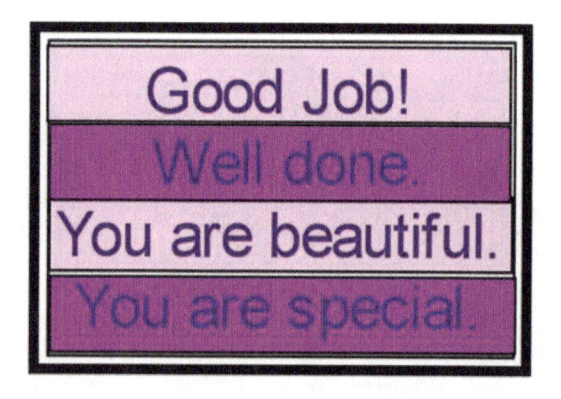

Good Job!
Well done.
You are beautiful.
You are special.

# 37

When you get angry, you don't make others' look bad – you make yourself look bad.

> Attitude is a little thing that makes a BIG DIFFERENCE.
> —Winston Churchill

# 38

Those who are not extremely opinionated don't anger easily. Just because it's your point of view, doesn't make it the only correct point of view.

> **I'm NOT opinionated**
>
> **I'm just always right!**

# 39

Anger is a prison. And you hold the key to freedom. Letting go of anger will unlock the gates to freedom.

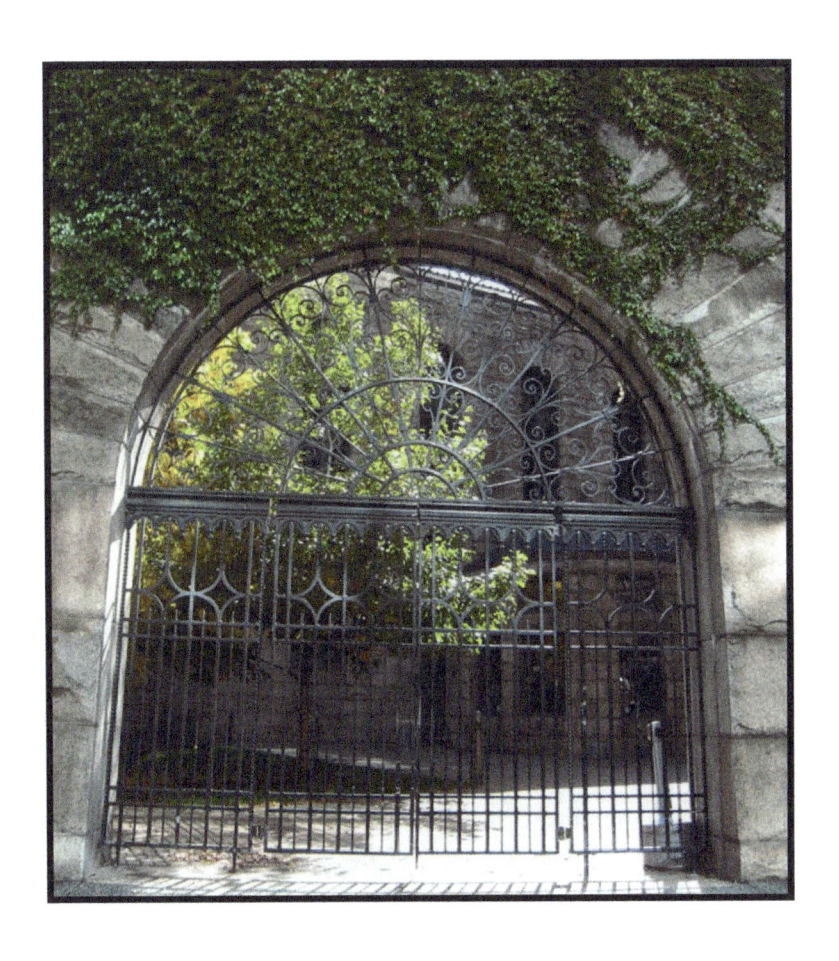

# 40

Assumptions are like termites: They eat away at your soul, destroy the core of all relationships and leave useless piles behind.

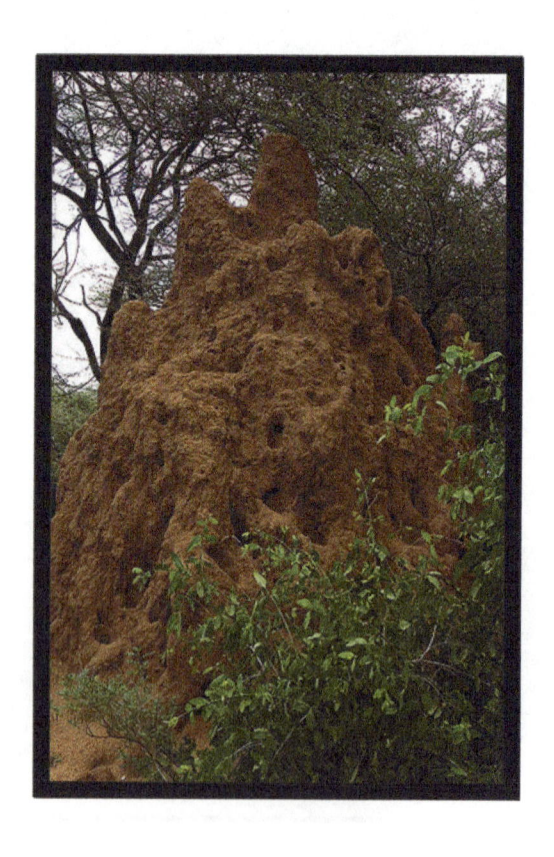

# 41

Turn anger into a four-letter word: LOVE.

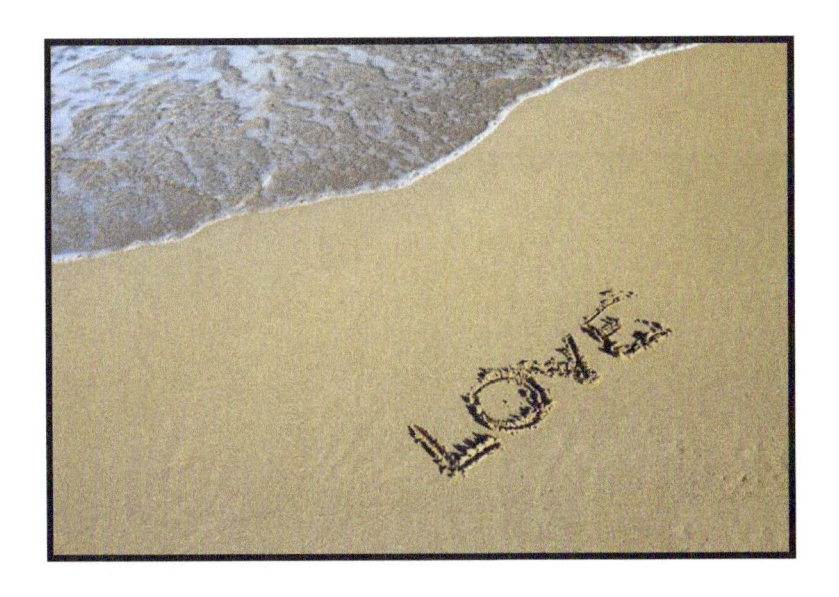

# 42

Angry thoughts are you reliving the past. Anger will prevent you from living a full and complete life. Living anger free will allow you to make the most of the life you have been given.

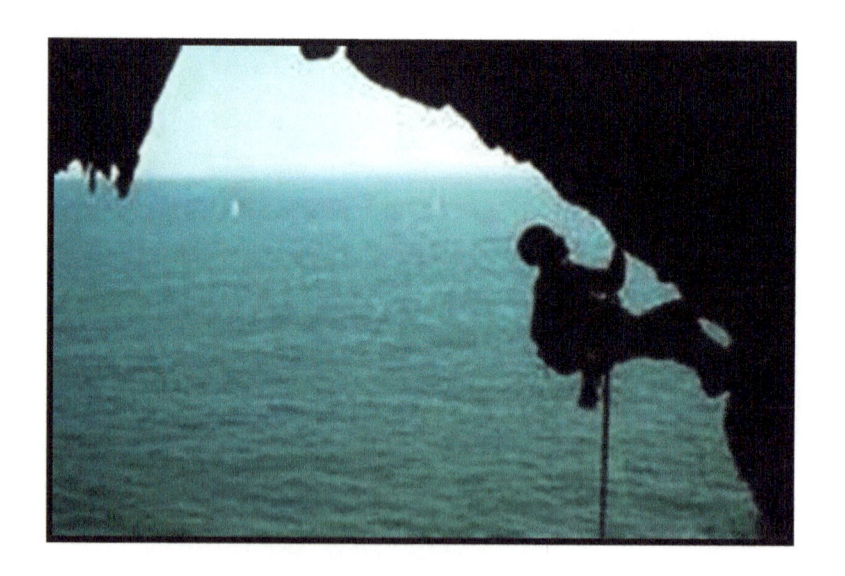

# 43

Those who cannot master their anger will become a slave to it. Ask yourself if you want to be the master or the slave. Don't allow anger to control your every move.

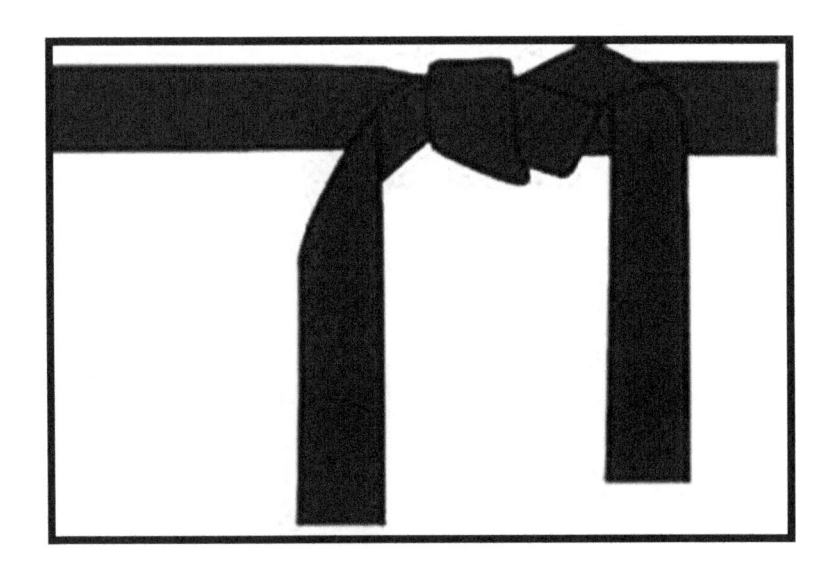

# 44

Remove any sense of entitlement. Believing you should always get what you want will create anger when you don't. Everyone is special, not just you.

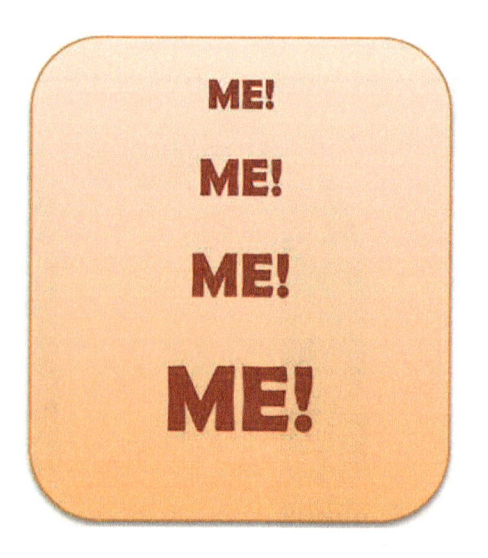

> **ME!**
> **ME!**
> **ME!**
> **ME!**

## 45

Anger causes isolation and social withdrawal. Remember to stay connected to friends, family and others on a daily basis. If you remain angry, you'll find yourself alone.

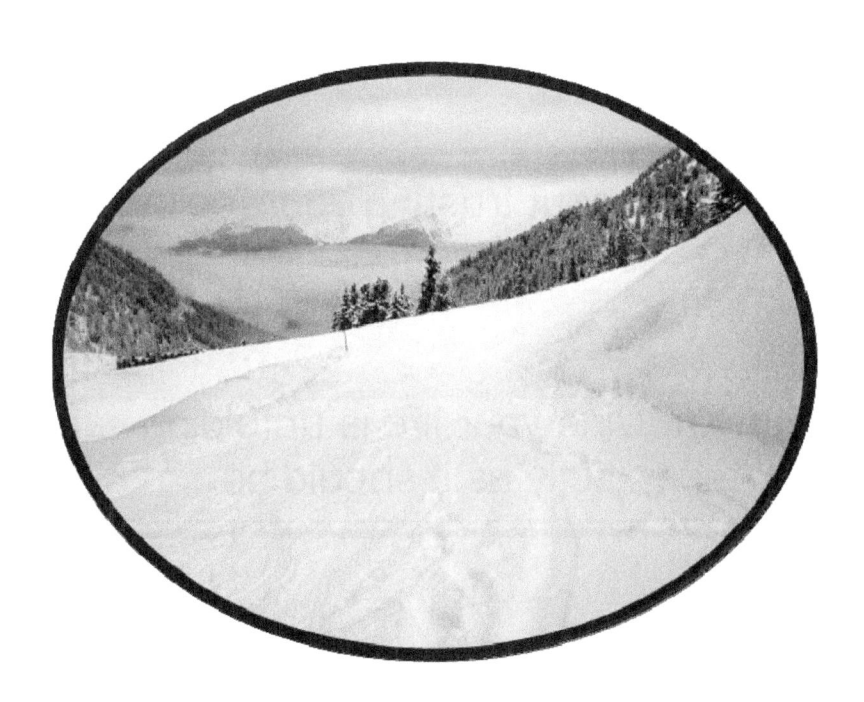

# 46

Worry and anxiety can lead to anger. Trust all is unfolding exactly the way it should be. Your anger will subside once you know there is nothing to be angry about. All is well.

| Life is about trusting your feelings and taking risks; |
|---|
| Trusting your hopes, not your fears, and |
| Knowing your life is unfolding exactly as it should be. |

# 47

When you catch yourself saying "That's not fair," remember fairness is subjective. What one person sees as fair, another person may see as an injustice.

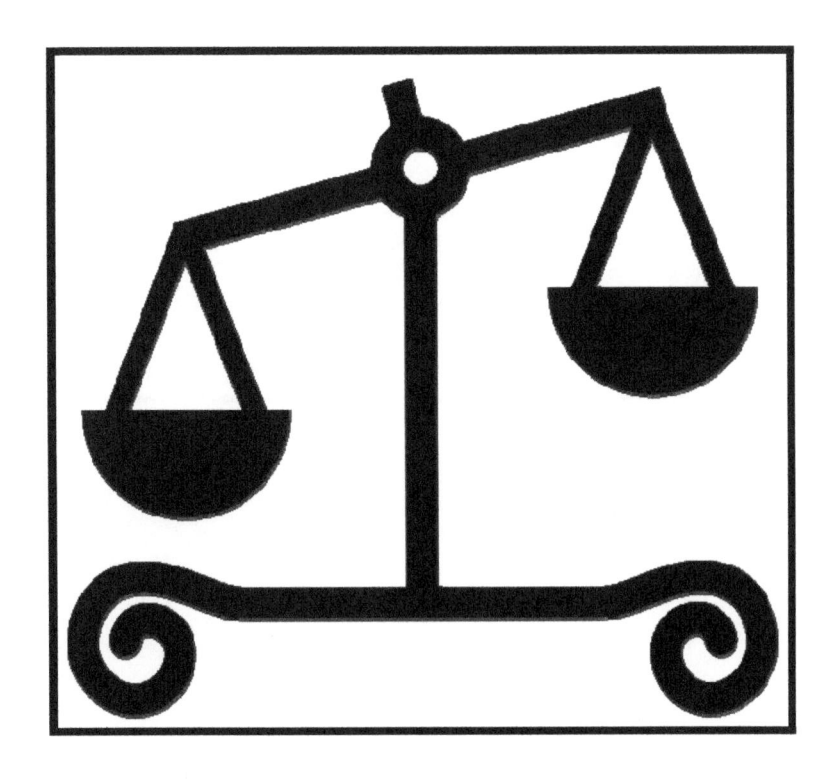

# 48

Know that you have the power within you to change. Your spirit is stronger than you think. No one is ordinary, everyone is extraordinary.

> What lies behind us and what lies before us are tiny matters... compared to what lies *within us.*
> -Ralph Waldo Emerson

# 49

Admit to your mistakes and learn to say "I'm sorry, please forgive me."

> **Forgiveness is not something we do for OTHER PEOPLE.**
>
> ★
>
> **We do it for OURSELVES - to GET WELL and MOVE ON.**

# 50

He who angers you conquers you.
—*Elizabeth Kenney*

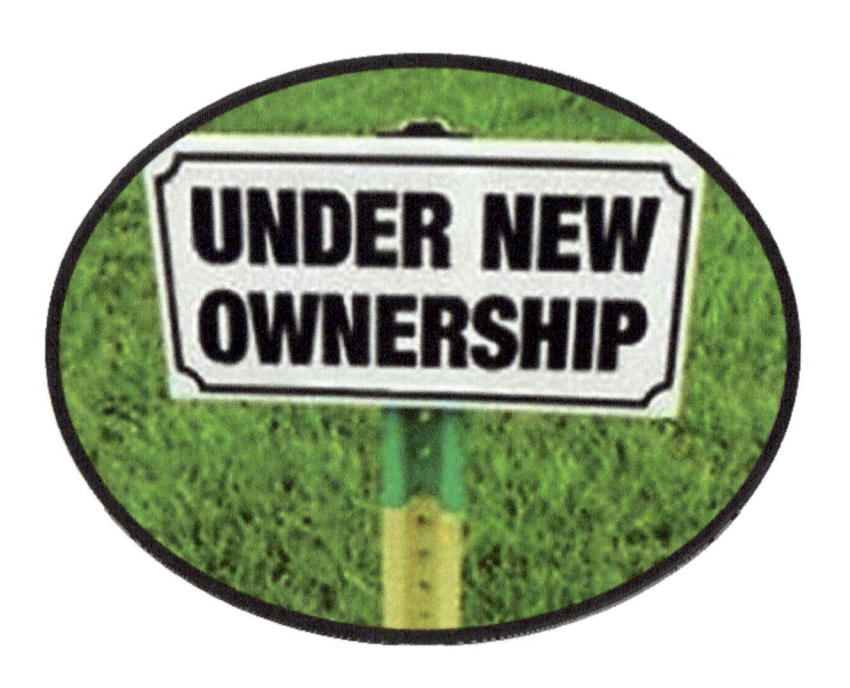

# 51

Anger is trash. When you get mad, you're polluting the environment. Keep your environment clean and beautiful.

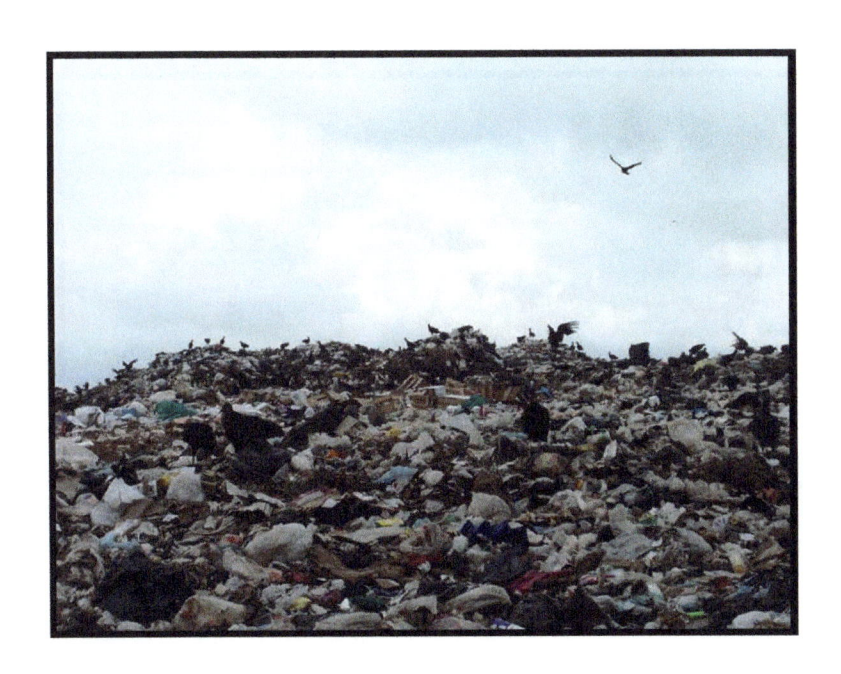

# 52

Anger is a trap. Don't get stuck in a trap. It will be harder to get out than it was to get in.

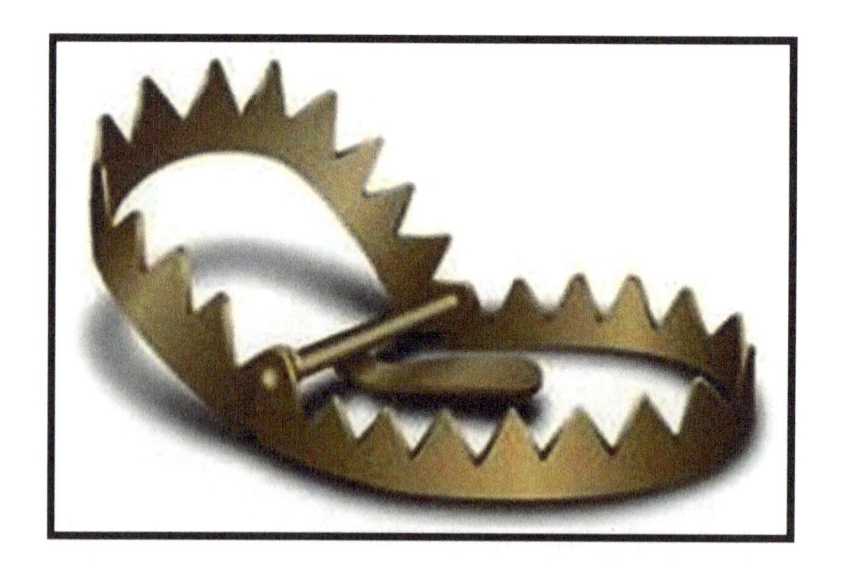

# 53

Asking for help is a sign of strength. Believing you won't ever need help is a sign of weakness. Learn to ask for help when you need it.

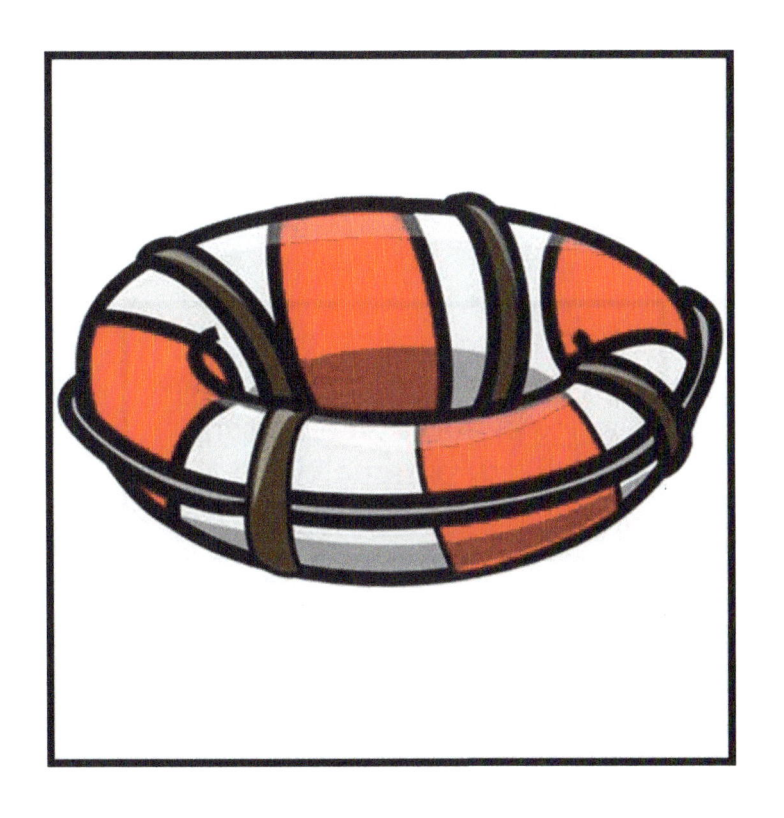

## 54

Take an online personality test. There are no right or wrong answers, and you will discover patterns in your behavior. When you find out what your strengths and weaknesses are, you can begin to bring about change.

www.similarminds.com
www.outofservice.com/bigfive/
www.personalityonline.com
www.yourpersonality.net
www.personalitytest.net

# 55

Anger erodes the soul. Peace makes the soul grow. Don't let your soul rot.

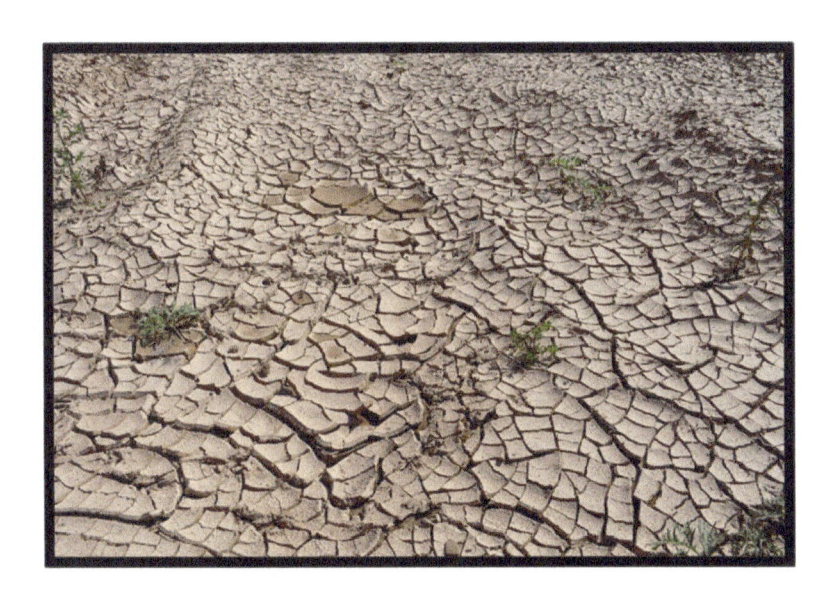

# 56

When you get angry, you become your own worst enemy. Avoid self-sabotage.

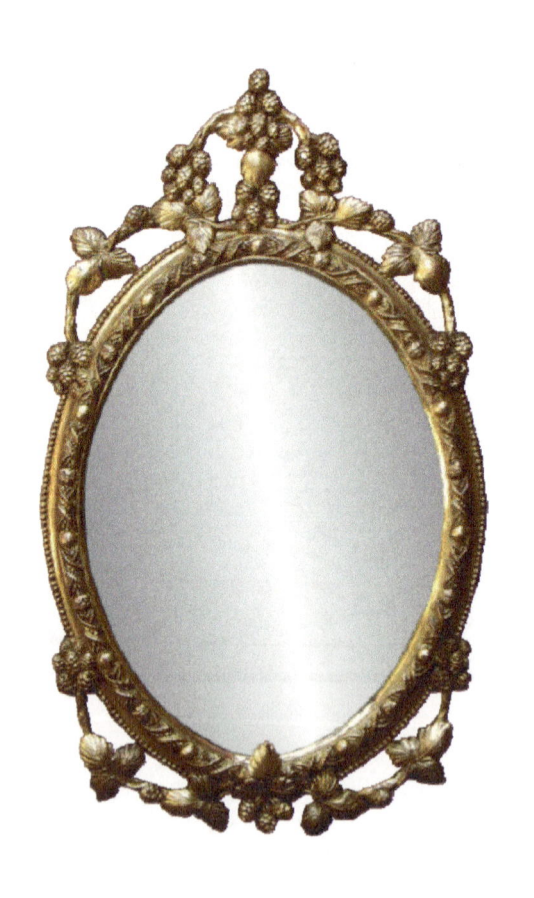

# 57

It is never beneficial to compare yourself to others. Learn to appreciate your unique talents, skills and circumstances. Everyone is beautiful just the way they are.

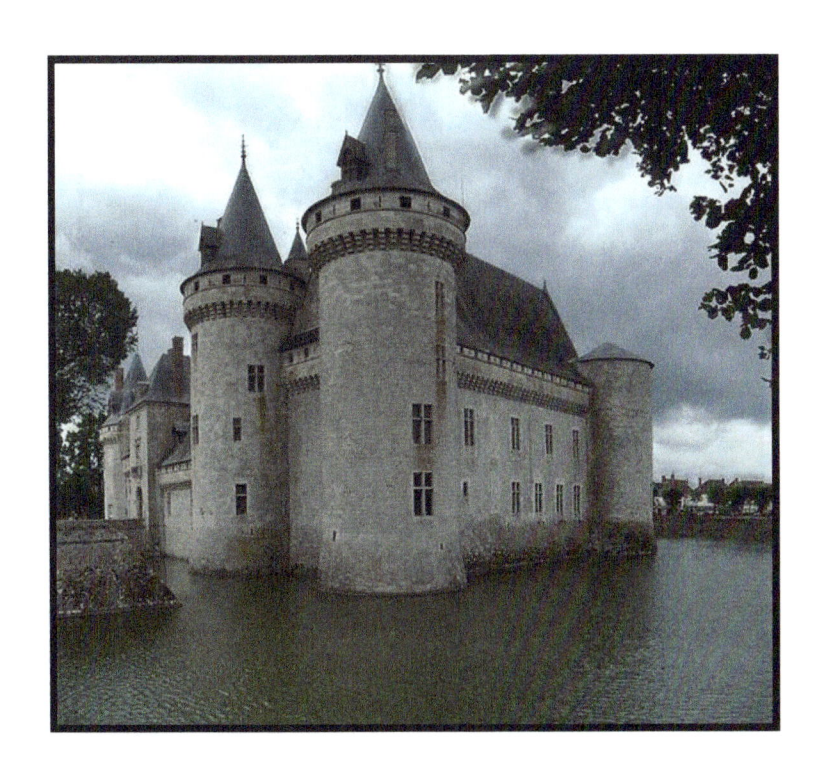

## 58

Whenever you are faced with a frustrating situation, use your creativity. Think outside the box by using your imagination and uniqueness.

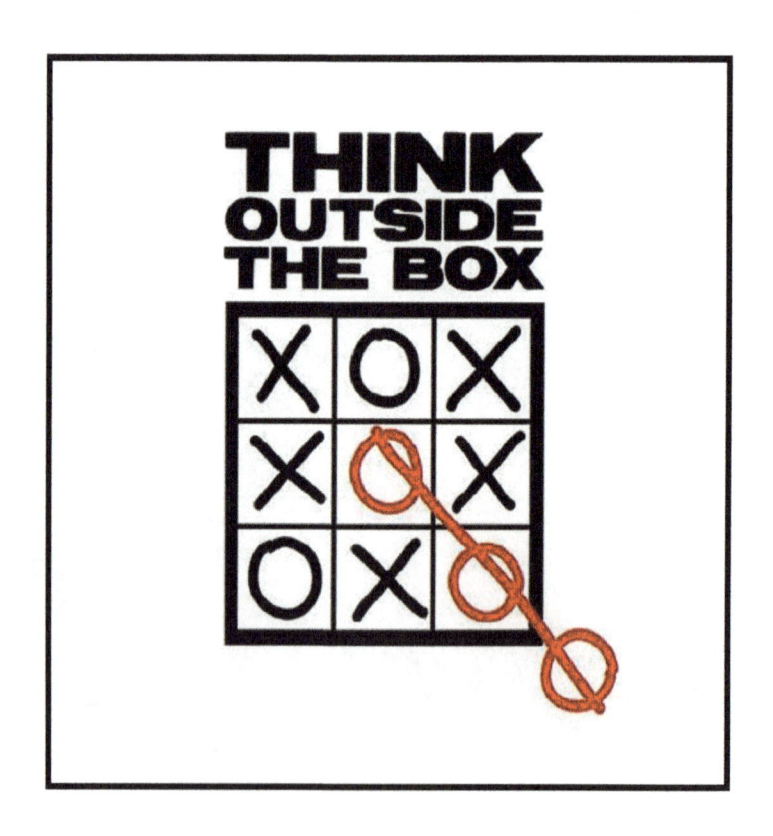

## 59

Think of others first. Anger presents itself when you are only thinking about yourself. To live anger-free, know that *you* are not the only person who matters.

> No act of kindness, no matter how small, is ever wasted.
> – Aesop

# 60

Know that you are no better than anyone else. We are all special and equal. Feelings of superiority cause anger.

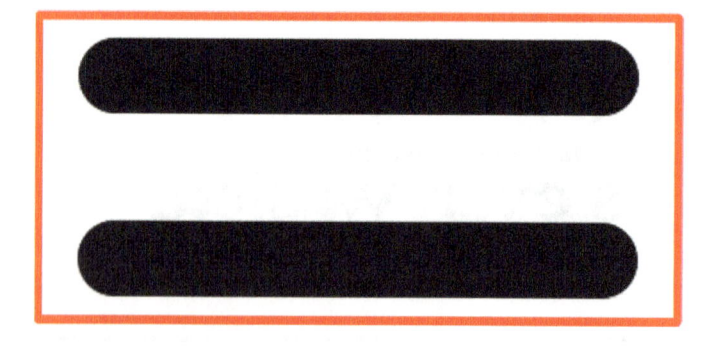

# 61

Being angry will not help a situation. Anger can only detract from an already poor situation.

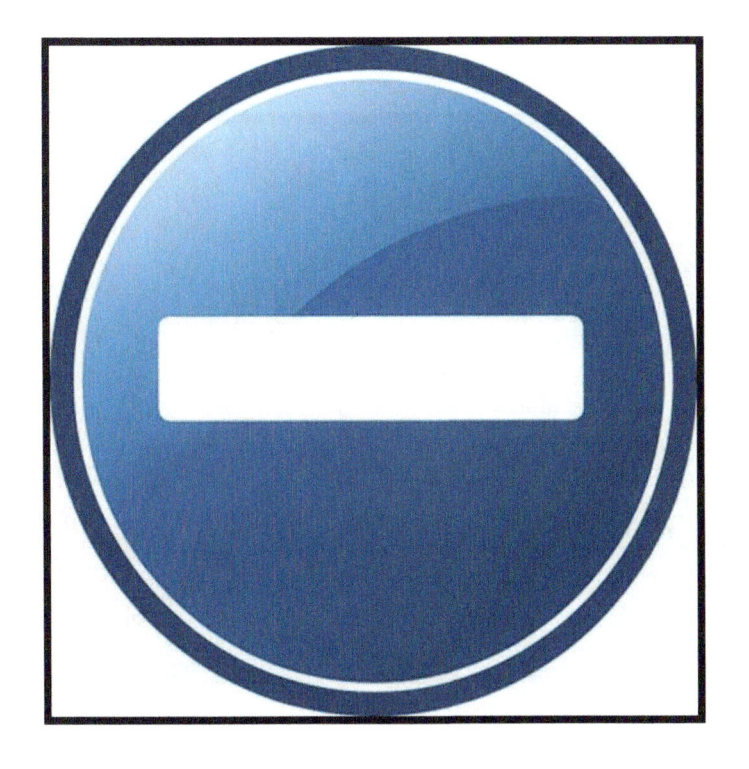

# 62

When you feel yourself getting mad, force yourself to smile instead. Smiling paves the way to laughter, and laughter truly is the best medicine.

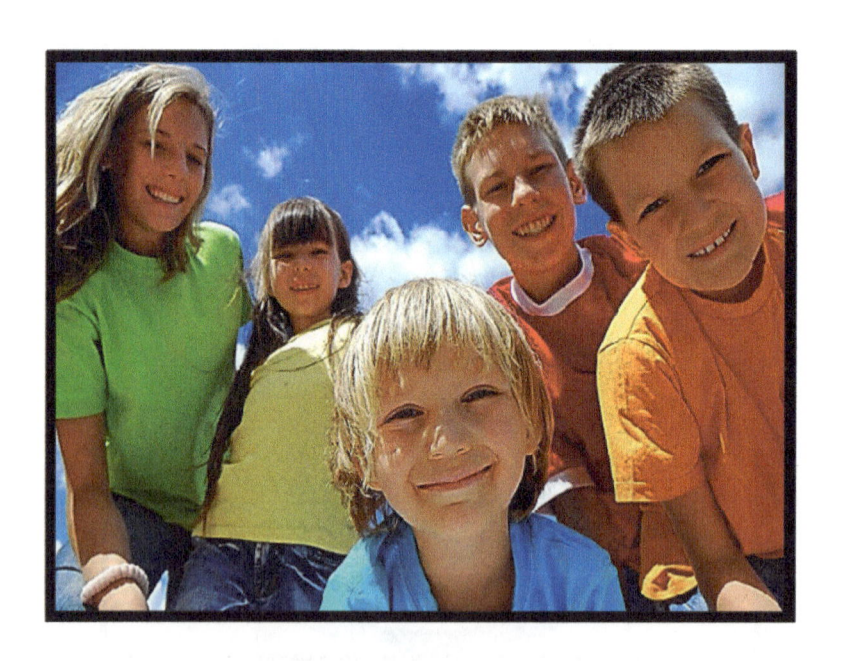

## 63

The second you feel angry, think of something that makes you happy — a song, flower, favorite snack, sport or pet.

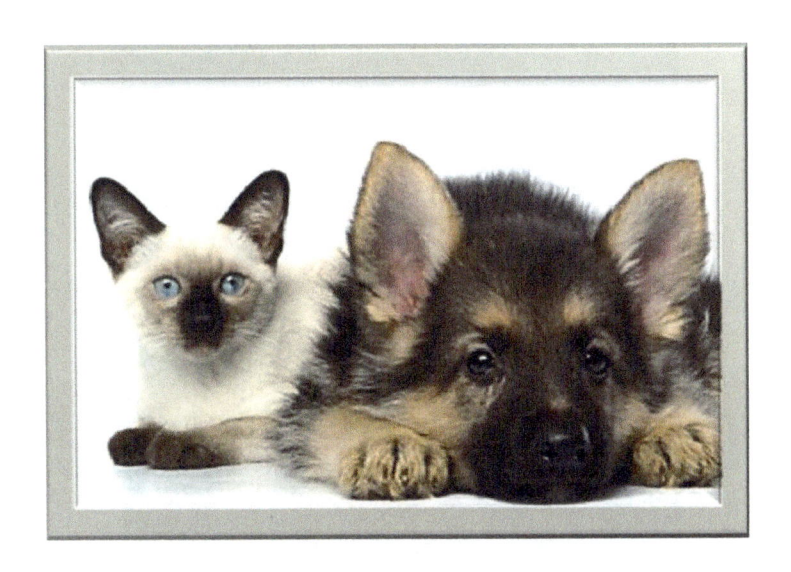

# 64

Think of all events as learning experiences. Instead of getting angry, look for room to grow and become better than you were. Strive to grow tall and strong.

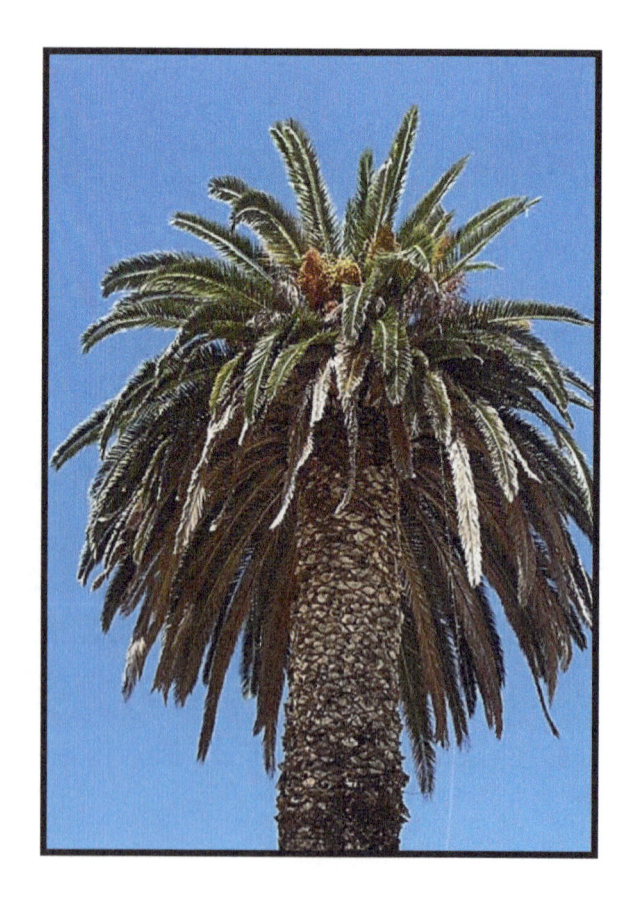

# 65

When you feel angry, encourage yourself to look at little things, for they are the things that matter most.

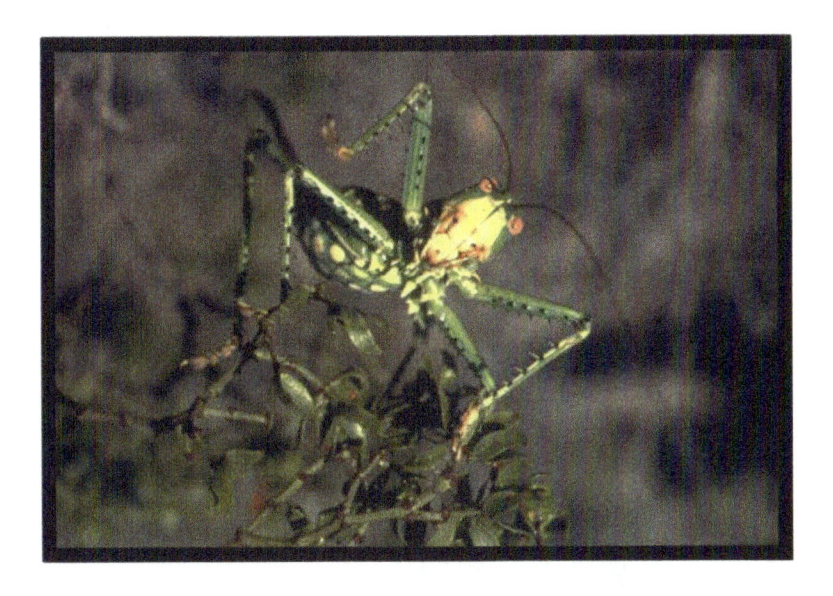

> Those who cannot feel the littleness in great things in themselves, are apt to overlook the greatness of little things in others.
>
> -*Kakuzo Okakura* (1862-1913)
>
> Japanese author and teaist

# 66

All things happen for a reason and a purpose. Luck, accidents and coincidences do not exist. Everything in your life fits together like pieces of a puzzle.

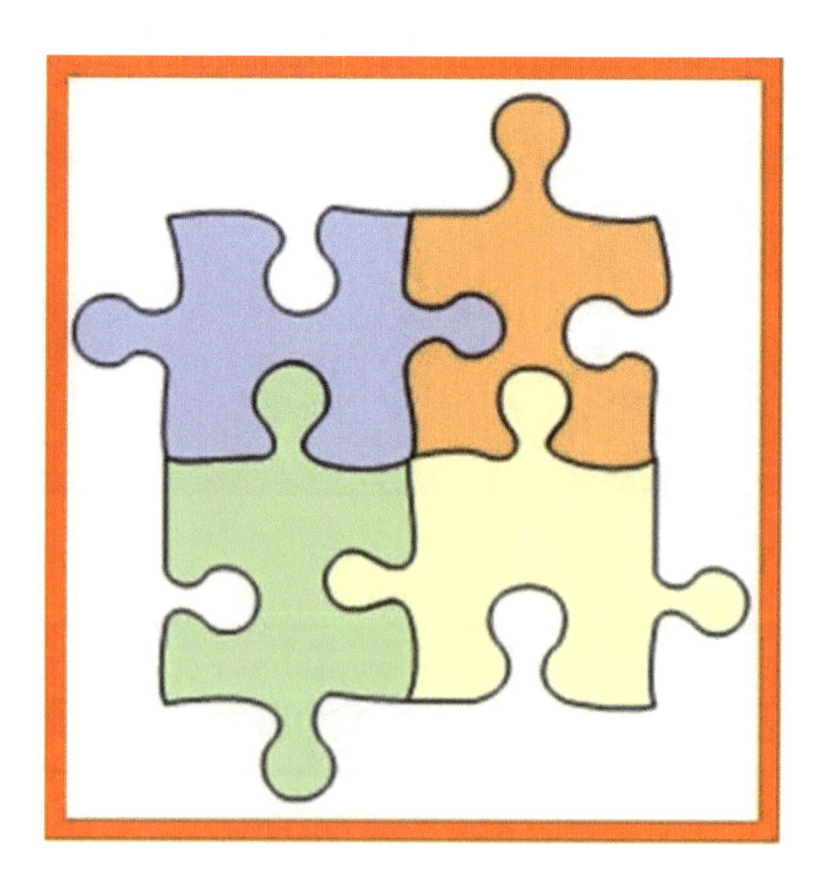

# 67

When turning in for the night, take time to think of all the things that are good in your life. Avoid dwelling on mistakes or what didn't go your way.

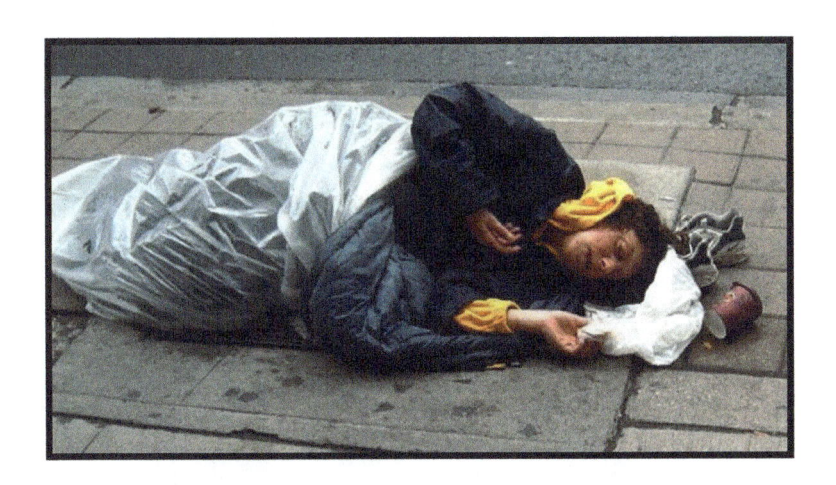

## 68

Know your limitations. Striving to accomplish too much can lead to frustration and anger.

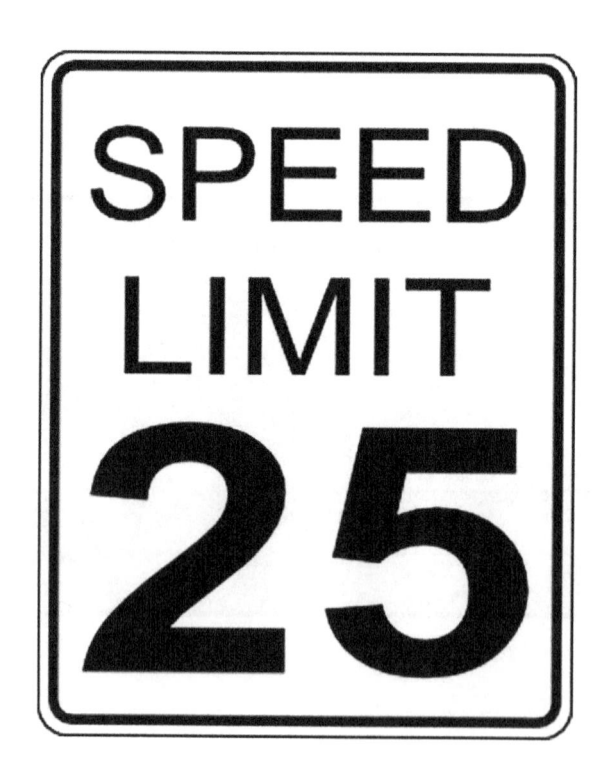

# 69

Not every day of your life will go as you planned. And that's okay. Go with the flow.

> *Everything will be okay in the end.*
> *If it's not okay,*
> *It's not the end.*
>
> -Author unknown

# 70

Anger may be caused by a misperception of reality. Rid yourself of unrealistic expectations.

> People who expect nothing
>
> will never be disappointed

# 71

Acceptance is essential. Accept all people and events for who and what they are.

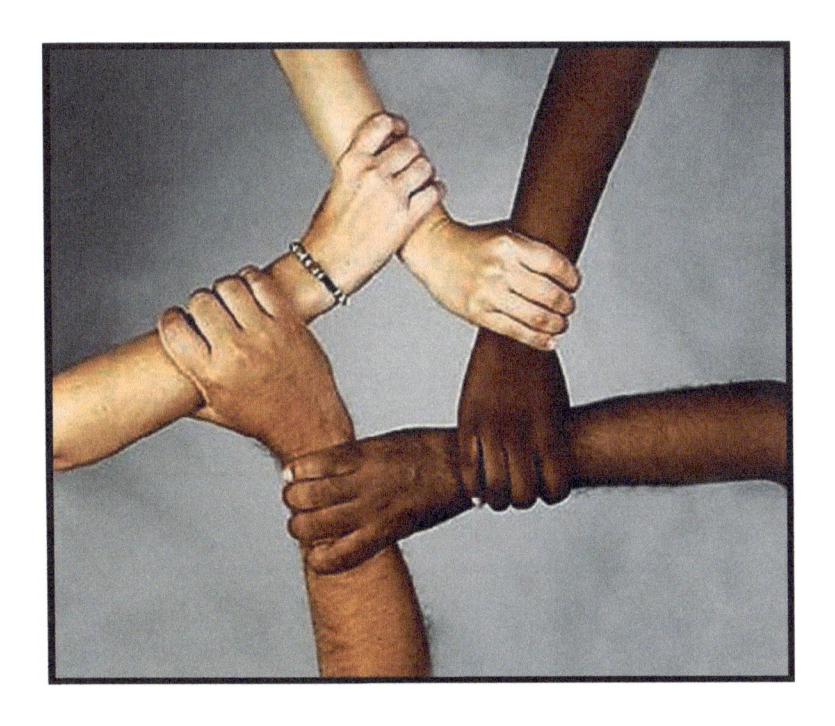

## 72

Know that blame is futile and only serves to fuel your anger.

> Blaming others doesn't make a person better than the one they are blaming. Blaming others is an excuse for not taking responsibility for your own actions.

# 73

"Holding on to anger is like grasping a hot coal with the intent of throwing it at someone else; you are the one who gets burned."

*–Gautama Buddha*
*Indian Spiritual Teacher*
*4th century* BCE

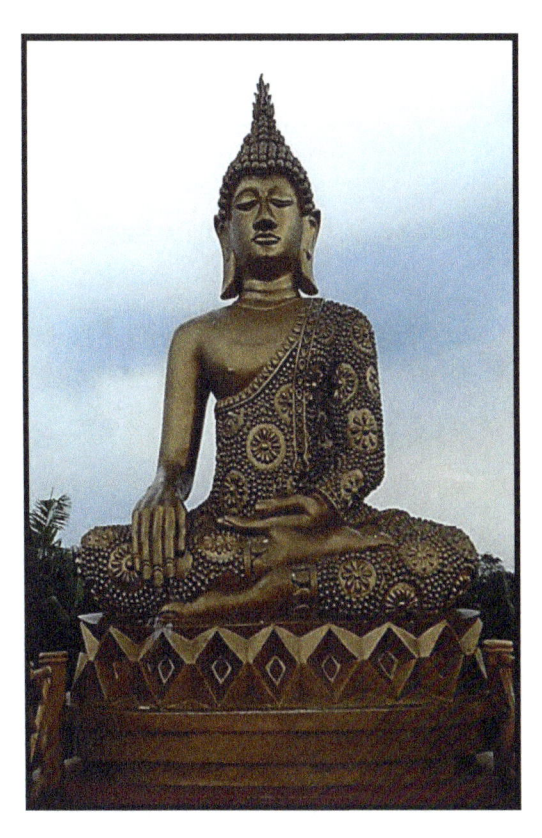

# 74

Avoid spanking or being physical with your children. Witnessing violence teaches children that violence is a solution.

> Violence is always the problem and never the solution.

# 75

Being angry is like living in your own personal hell. Don't put yourself in hell.

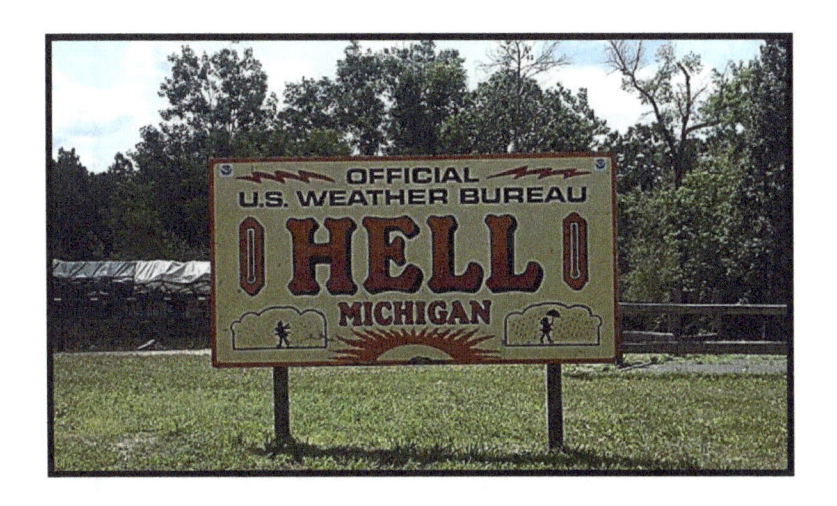

## 76

Anxiety can contribute to angry thoughts. Find ways on a daily basis to reduce your stress. Avoid worry; it won't make the situation any better.

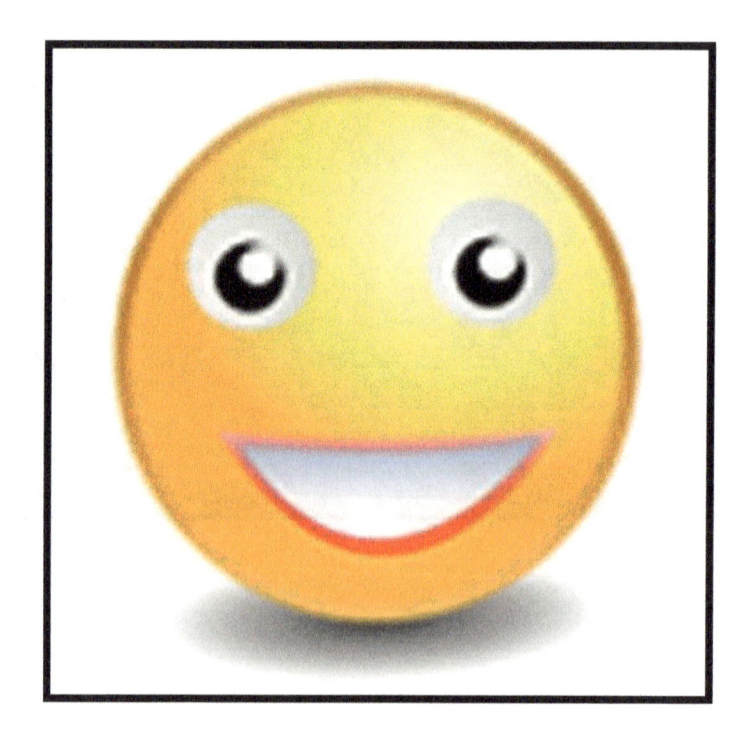

# 77

Anger leads to more anger. Love leads to more love.

"Love is life. Love is God. All, everything that I understand, I understand only because I love. Everything is, everything exists, only because I love. Everything is united by it alone."

*–Leo Nikolayevich Tolstoy, Russian Writer and Poet, 1828 – 1910*

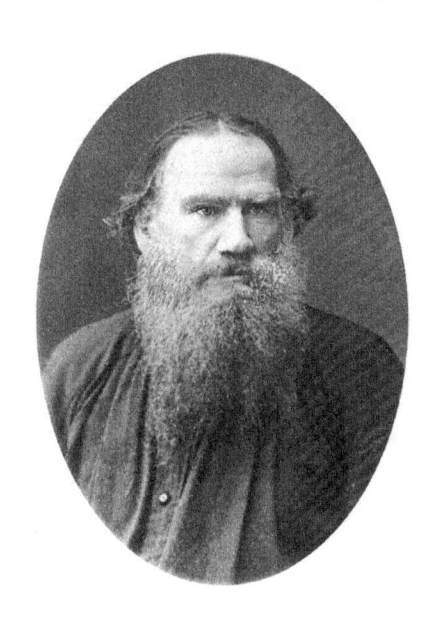

# 78

When you feel angry, avoid speaking. Just sit in silence, close your eyes and think of why you feel helpless. Then take steps to turn that feeling around.

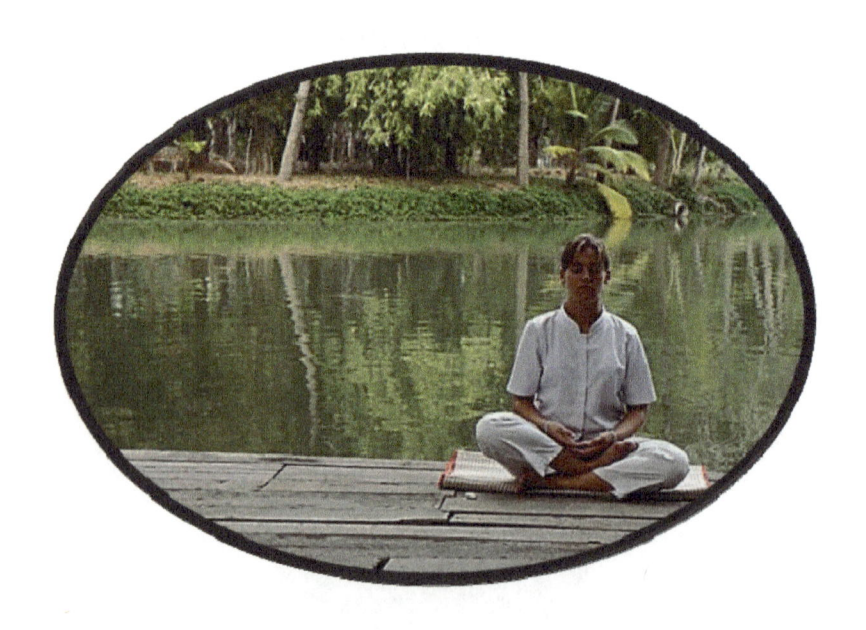

# 79

No one is a mind reader. To believe you know the intent of other people's actions without asking them will only create angry feelings.

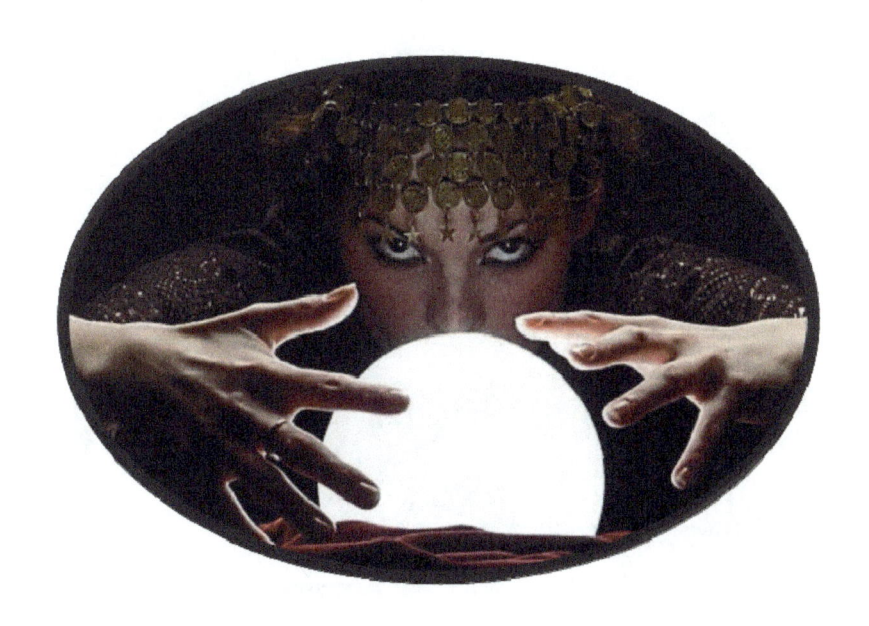

# 80

You won't always get what you want. And that's okay. Embrace what you did receive instead of hating it.

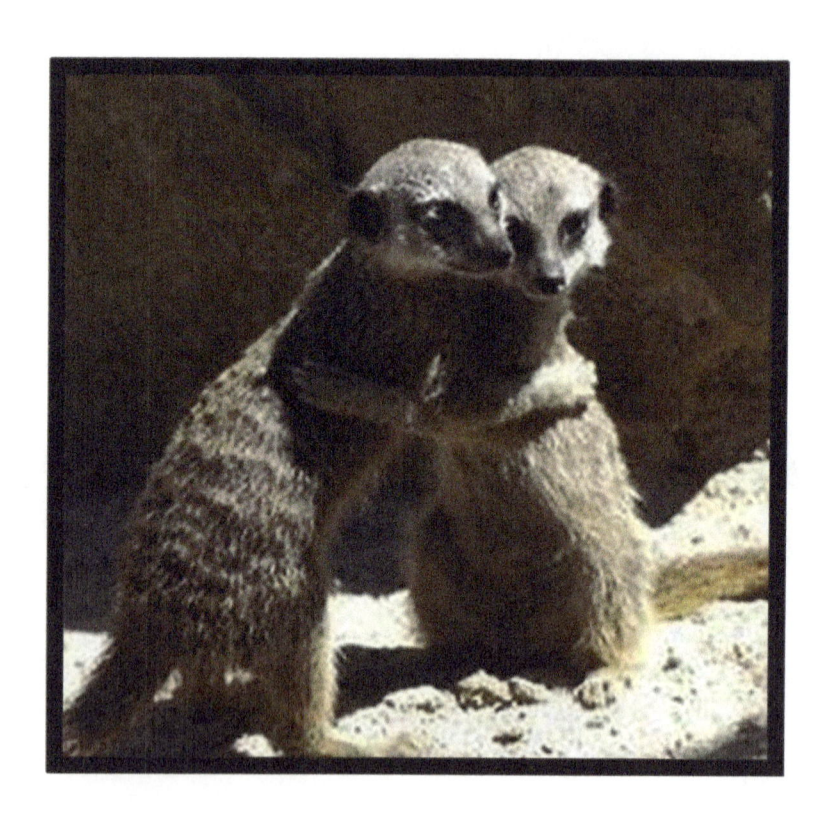

# 81

Remember, everyone does things differently. When you expect others to be exactly like you, you are making yourself mad over that which will never be.

> Great minds do not think alike.
>
> Great minds think differently.

# 82

No one makes you mad. *You* allow yourself to get mad over the actions of others. Take back your power by controlling your anger.

> Each morning we are born again. What we do today is what matters most.
>
> —Buddha

## 83

Try to see both sides of the coin so you can understand someone else's position. Understanding brings tolerance, and tolerance combats anger.

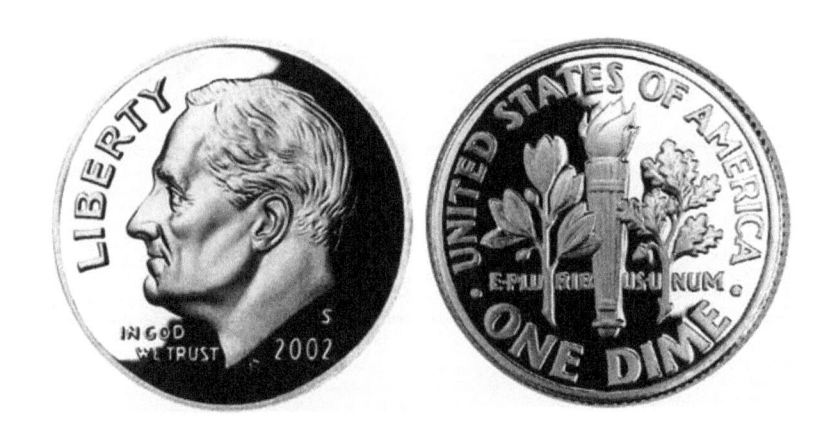

# 84

Remember this quote from the Bible: "Do unto others as you would have them do unto you."

*–Luke 6:31*

> Kindness is never wrong.
> Even when others are not
> kind in return.

# 85

Anger is a poison. The only way to get the poison out is to let go of the anger. Avoid ingesting poison – don't let anything bother you.

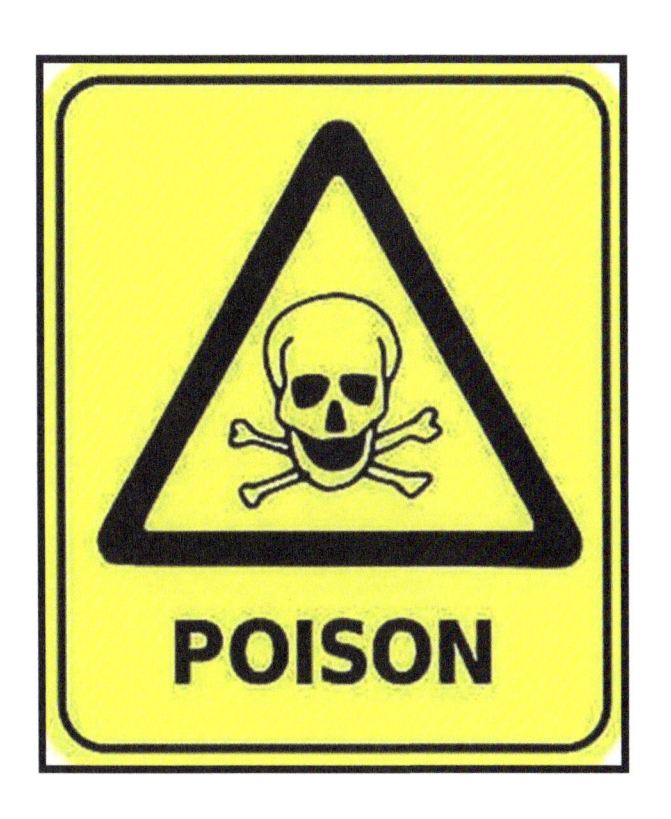

# 86

We all have to do things we don't want to do. Do the right thing, even if it will be unpleasant or difficult.

> Integrity is doing the right thing even when no one is watching.

# 87

Never give up hope. Hope takes away fear and anger.

> The most common way people give up their power is by thinking they don't have any.
> -Alice Walker
> Author of the Color Purple

# 88

Anger causes revengeful thoughts, and revenge is never the proper reaction to any situation.

*An eye for an eye makes the whole world blind.*
*- Mahatma Gandhi*

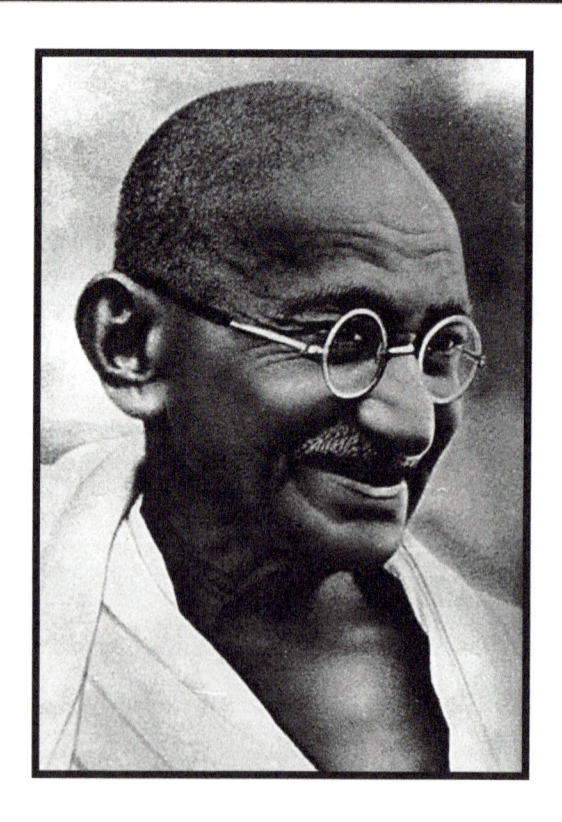

# 89

Look within and let go of whatever is bothering you. Remember, there are three types of business: yours, God's and other people's. If it's not your business, let it go.

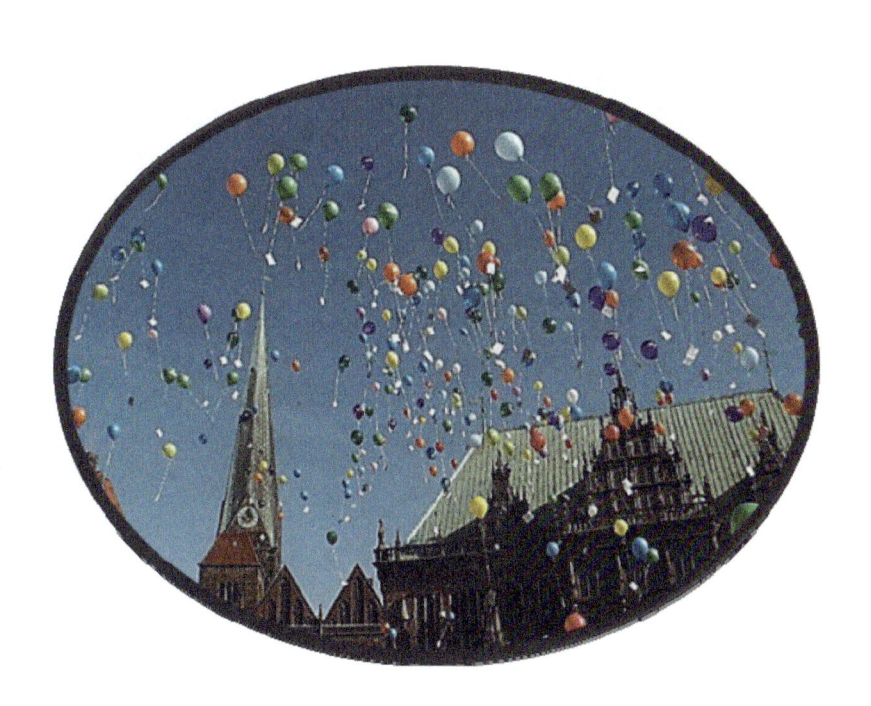

## 90

Like a tornado, anger destroys. It destroys souls, friendships, relationships, marriages and a person's self-esteem.

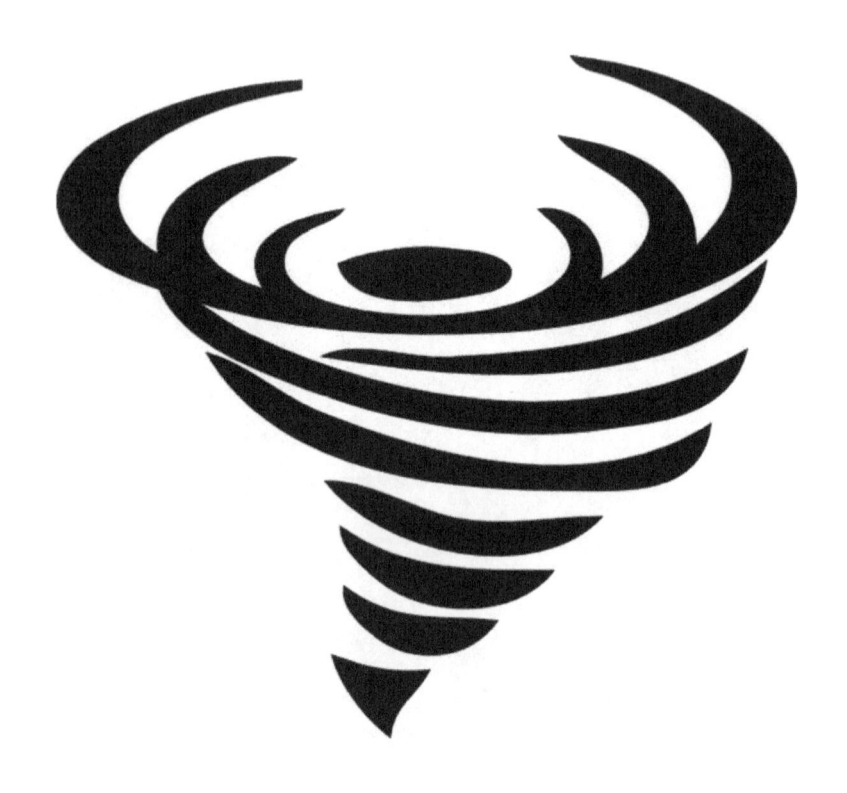

# 91

If you feel your anger is beyond your control, seek help from a mental health professional. Chemical imbalances in the brain may produce uncontrollable anger.

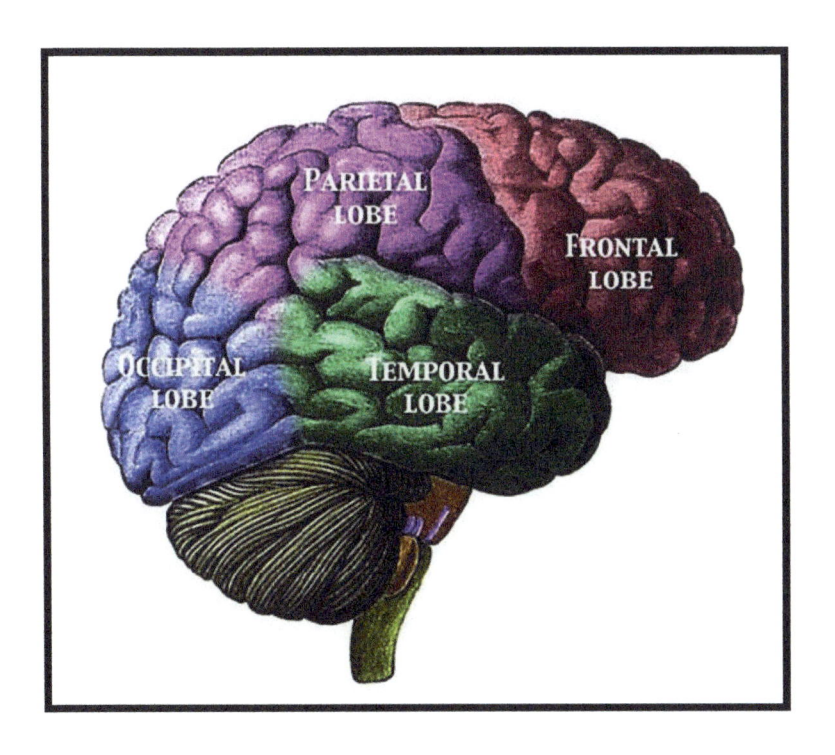

# 92

Work daily to put ANGER out of your life.

| A | anxiety |
|---|---|
| N | narcissism |
| G | greed |
| E | entitlement |
| R | resentment |

# 93

You cannot fully understand and show compassion for others when you are angry.

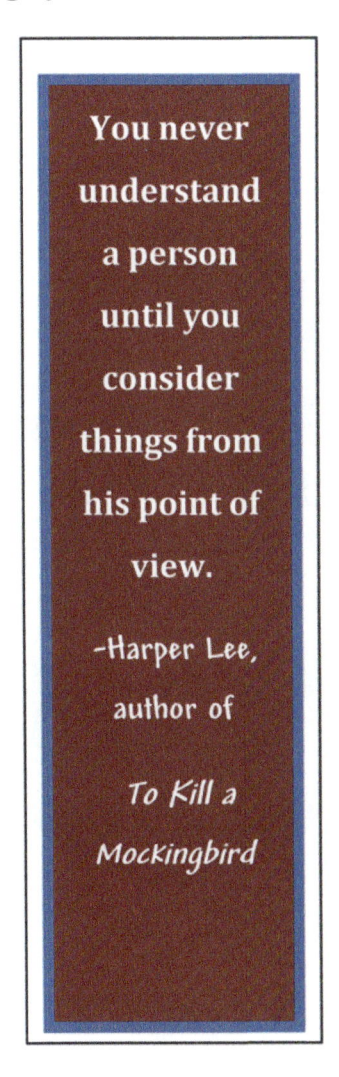

> You never understand a person until you consider things from his point of view.
>
> –Harper Lee, author of
>
> *To Kill a Mockingbird*

# 94

"Whatever is begun in anger ends in shame."

*–Benjamin Franklin*
*Philosopher and Statesman*
*1706–1790*

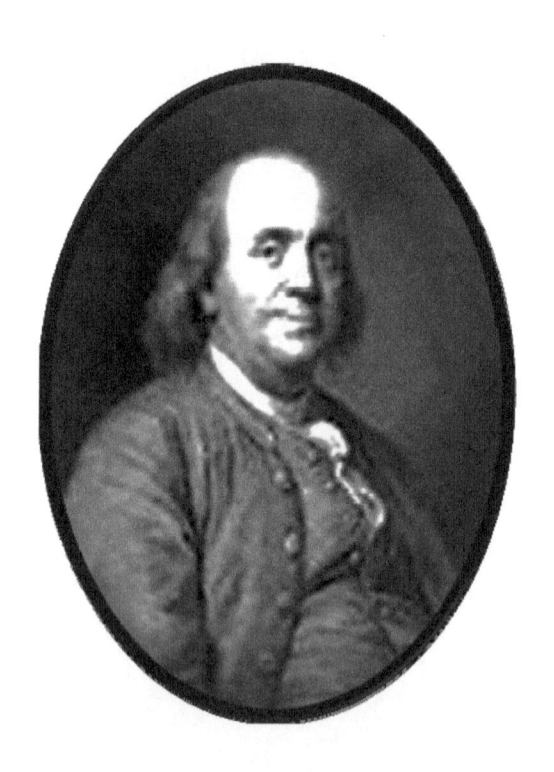

# 95

Two wrongs don't make a right. When you get angry at someone for getting angry at you, the issue still remains unresolved.

wrong ✚ wrong = ~~right~~ wrong

# 96
## Turn ANGER into PEACE.

**P** urpose

**E** nrichment

**A** dmiration

**C** almness

**E** mpathy

## 97

Jealousy is a worthless emotion. It will only cause anger and self-hatred.

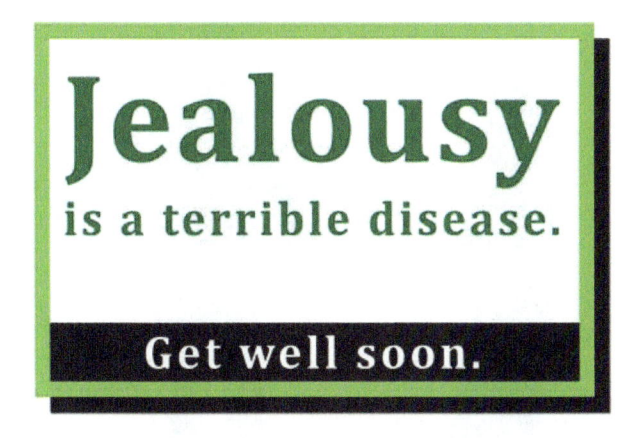

**Jealousy is a terrible disease. Get well soon.**

## 98

Talk to your parents, friend, spouse or counselor. While talking out your problems, you may find a solution or an alternative way of doing things. That, in turn, will help relieve anger.

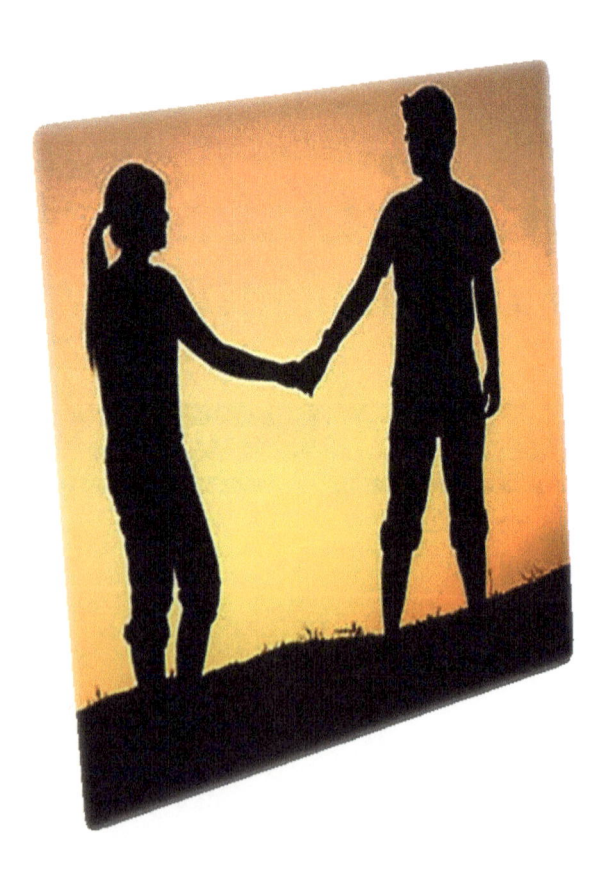

## 99

Buried beneath anger is love and contentment. Be willing to do whatever it takes to feel love, harmony and peace.

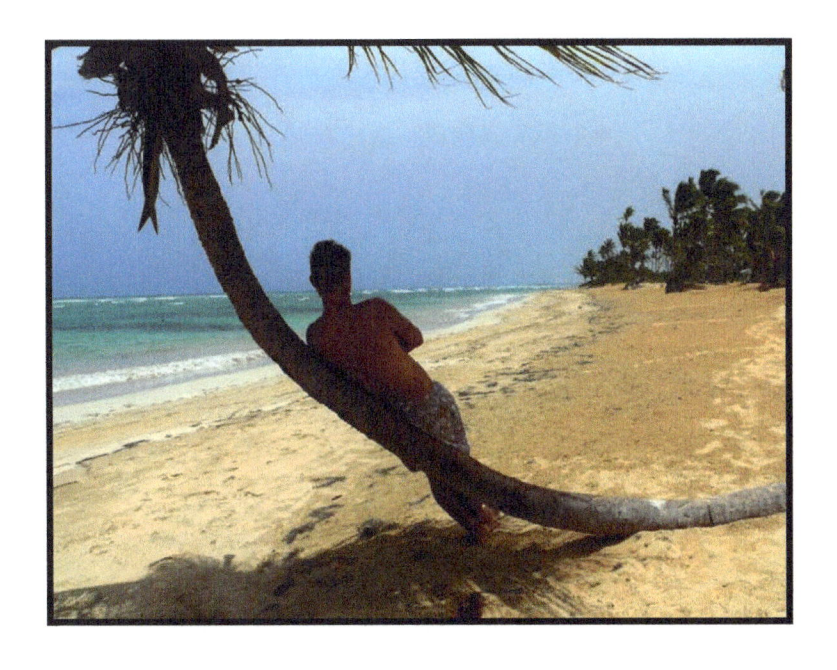

## 100

Avoid complaining. The more you complain, the angrier you will be. And the situation will still not have changed. Seek to find a solution instead.

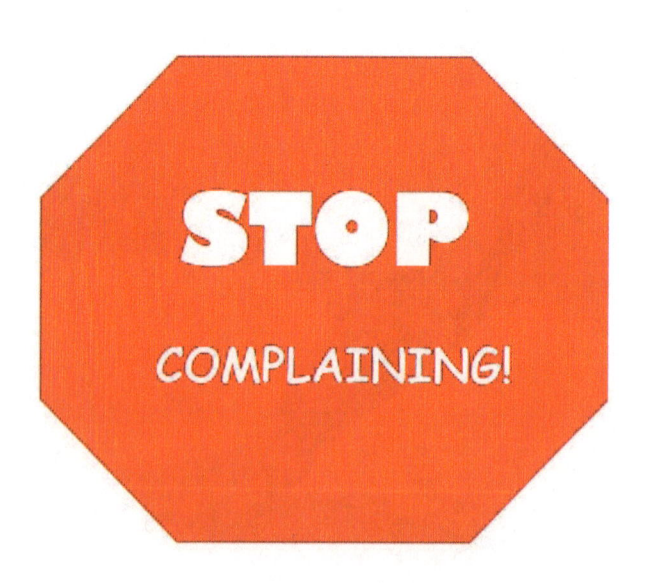

## 101

Surrender. Give up your need for control. Let all things happen without trying to make them happen your way.

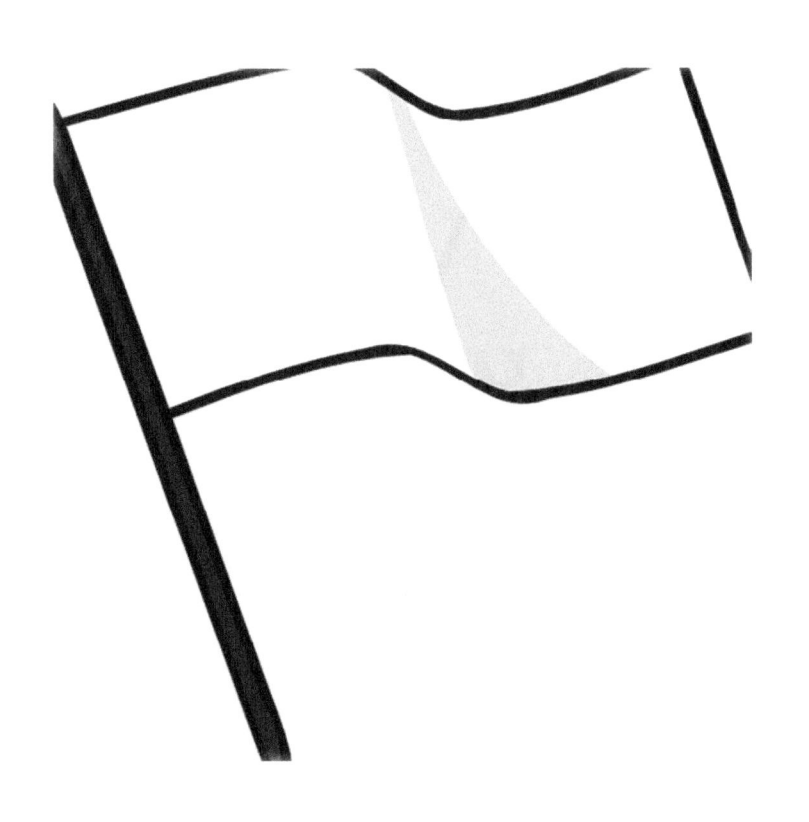

## 102

Go one day without getting angry. Then another and then another. The longer you are anger free, the less likely you are to get upset again.

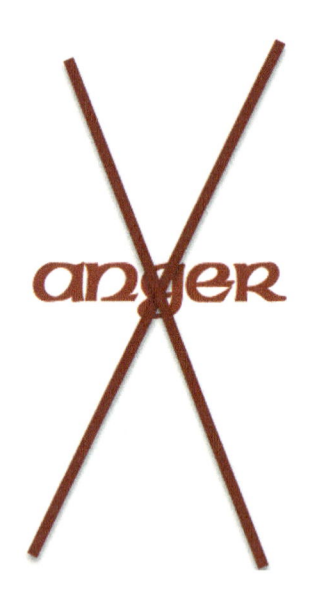

# 103

Practice unconditional love. Love the unique, unusual and uncommon, even if you don't understand them.

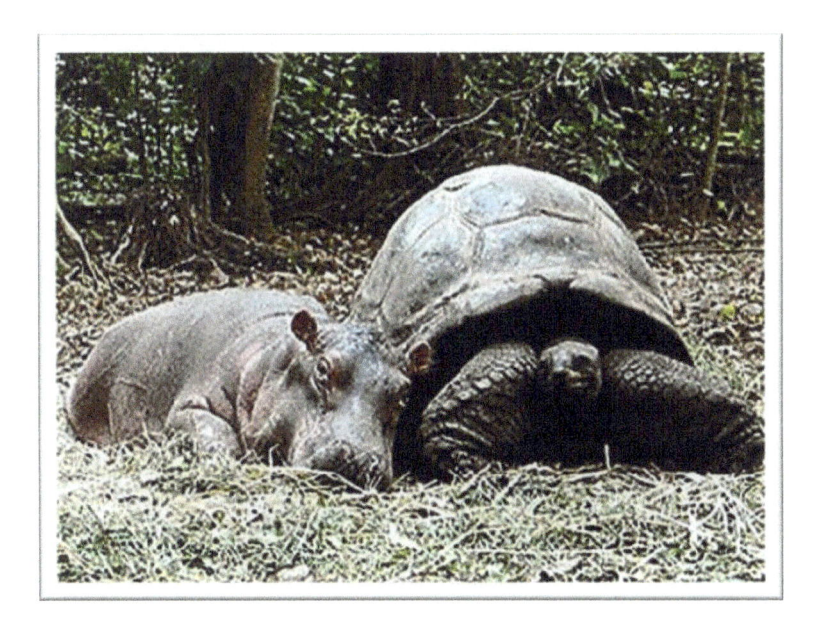

# 104

Don't expect circumstances to adapt to you. Learn to adapt to the circumstances that arise before you.

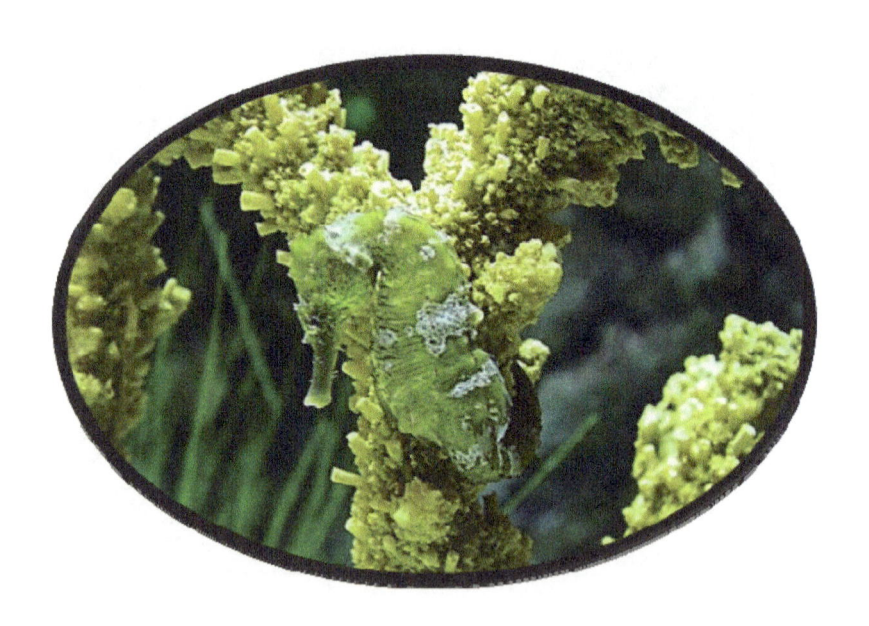

# Prayers

## I'm Angry, God

I'm angry, God,

Help me to understand my feelings.

Help me to see the other person's side of things.

Help me to control my words and my actions.

Help me to look for a solution to the problem that won't hurt anyone – most of all, me.

Amen

*–Ezekiel 7*

## The Serenity Prayer

GOD, grant me the serenity to accept the things I cannot change, courage to change the things I can and the wisdom to know the difference.

Living one day at a time; enjoying one moment at a time; accepting hardship as the pathway to peace. Taking, as He did, this sinful world as it is, not as I would have it.

Trusting that He will make all things right if I surrender to His Will. That I may be reasonably happy in this life and supremely happy with Him forever in the next.

Amen

*–Karl Paul Reinhold Niebuhr*
*Lutheran Pastor, 1926*

## Make Me a Channel of Thy Peace

Lord, make me a channel of thy peace.
That where there is hatred I may bring love,
That where there is wrong, I may bring the spirit of forgiveness,
That where there is discord, I may bring harmony,
That where there is error I may bring truth,
That where there is doubt I may bring faith,
That where there is despair I may bring hope,
That where there are shadows I may bring light,
That where there is sadness I may bring joy.
Lord, grant that I may seek rather to comfort than to be comforted,
To understand than to be understood,
To love than to be loved,
For it is by forgetting self that one finds.
It is by forgiving that one is forgiven,
it is by dying that one awakens to eternal life.
Amen

*–Version of the Prayer of Saint Francis
Delivered by Mother Teresa
to the United Nations, 1985*

## Related Resources

Dyer, Wayne. 1993. *Everyday Wisdom.* Carlsbad, CA: Hay House.

Dyer, Wayne. 1995. *101 Ways to Transform Your Life.* Carlsbad, CA: Hay House.

Dyer, Wayne. 2006. *Inspiration: Your Ultimate Calling.* Carlsbad, CA: Hay House.

Shimoff, Marci. 2008. *Happy for No Reason: 7 Steps to Being Happy from the Inside Out.* Minnetonka, MN: Learning Strategies Corp.

Tzu, Lao. 6th Century BCE. *Tao Te Ching.*

# About the Author

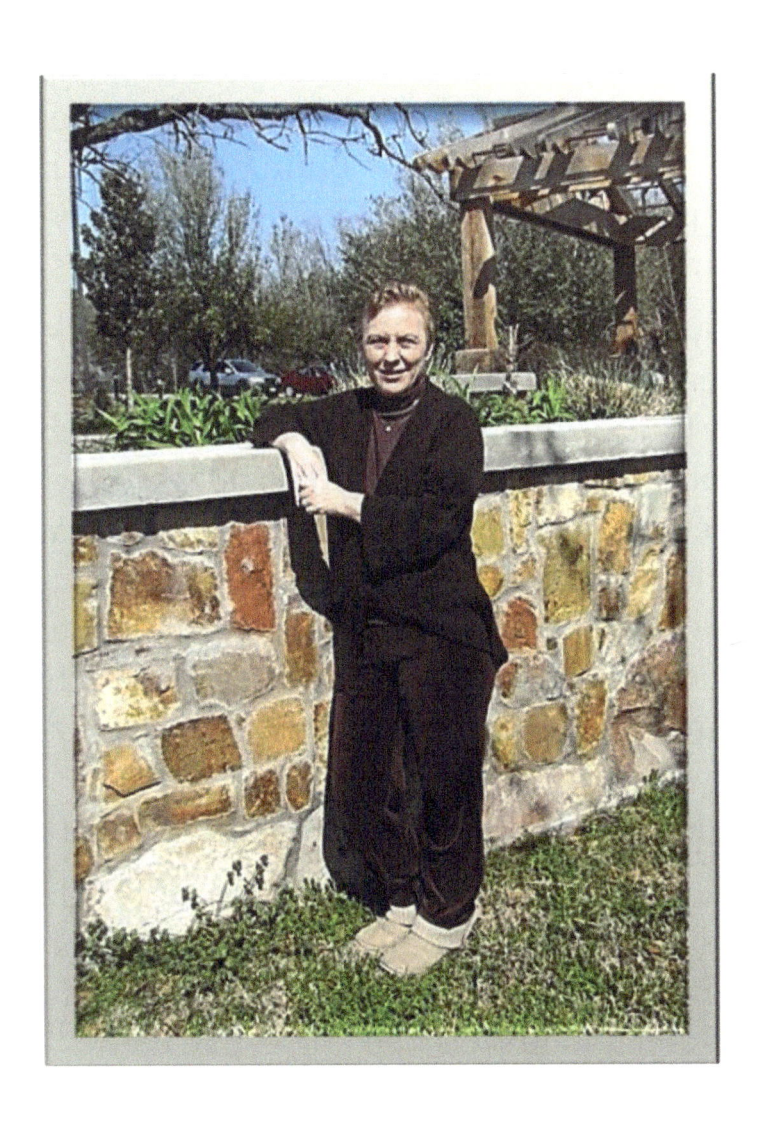

Robyn Wheeler was diagnosed with a form of neurotic depression called dysthymic disorder in 2010, at 44 years of age. Before her diagnosis, she struggled with chronic anger, anxiety and frustration. Now, on a daily regimen of medication regulating the chemical imbalance in her brain, most of her symptoms are gone or have improved dramatically, including her chronic anger.

Robyn wrote her first book, *Born Mad*, to help others suffering from dysthymic disorder and uncontrollable anger. *Born Mad* is a true account of Robyn's everyday struggles with anger and anxiety, and how she eventually found peace and happiness. She is the owner of Born Mad, LLC, a Texas-based company dedicated to creating awareness for dysthymic disorder and helping others who suffer from mental illness.

Robyn is currently a newspaper reporter, as well as an author and inspirational public speaker for her company regarding how people can conquer anger and why forgiveness is mandatory for an anger-free life.

She also teaches children how to create gratitude journals, say daily affirmations and turn harmful thinking into helpful thinking.

Robyn is a proud member of the National Alliance on Mental Illness (NAMI), National Association of Professional Women (NAPW), Worldwide Who's Who and the National association of the Self-Employed (NASE).

She is a Certified Family-to-Family Education Instructor for the NAMI Kaufman Chapter in Texas, and she was named 2012 Professional Woman of the Year by NAPW and 2012 Professional of the Year in Writing and Editing from Worldwide Who's Who.

Robyn and *Born Mad* are receiving 5-star ratings on Amazon and have appeared on numerous television, radio, newspaper, magazine and Web outlets, including Fox, NBC, *The Monitor of Cedar Creek Lake*, *The Double Ds in the Morning*, *Dresser After Dark*, *Your Family Health*, *The Mary Jones Show* and *Real Coaching Radio Network*.

CPSIA information can be obtained at www.ICGtesting.com
Printed in the USA
LVOW020538010213

318191LV00006B/12/P

9 780615 694504